Essentials of
Medical Management
Second Edition

edited by Wesley Curry and Barbara J. Linney, MA

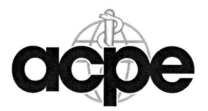

American College of Physician Executives
400 North Ashley Drive • Suite 400
Tampa, Florida 33602

ISBN: 0-9787306-4
Library of Congress Card Number: 2011937402
Printed in the United States of America

Contents

Chapter 1

Twenty-five Years as a Physician Executive

The Brief Memoirs of a "Suit"

by Robert Klint, MD, MHA

Mother cried when I told her. Well, maybe not cried, perhaps just a teary eyed gasp. It took such a long time to get here, to become a real doctor, and now this? My parents were delighted on my graduation from Brown University, although I thought I saw as much relief as delight. At graduation from medical school, it was all pride; "my son, the doctor" emerged in cap and gown. Soon there would be an office, patients, income, and more promise. And now I was "throwing it all away" to go into management, a seemingly far more pedestrian occupation from which one could be fired, demoted, or mergered out of existence, unlike medicine with its public high regard and nearly guaranteed employment. No, my decision to leave eight years of practice as a pediatric cardiologist and join the ranks of "administration" did not go particularly well at home.

Physicians on my medical staff were more blasé. When Hans Vandmeter, our chairman of medicine, heard of my decision, he simply said, "ve vill miss you." He ran his department as if it were a Prussian infantry division. To him, my leaving medicine and joining "them" was only slightly less outrageous than desertion. "Suits," those amorphous administrative people, who were frequently unknown and generally viewed as obstructive to the more humanitarian goals of the medical staff, could only be a backwater in the mainstream of medical care.

Of course there were well-wishers, clinicians who saw that their views and their patients' wishes just might have a better forum with a physician among the "suits." A few others, futurists mostly, saw a natural progression of responsibilities; the natural next career predicted in John Naisbitt's *Megatrends,*[1] perhaps a trend of the future. And a very few, mostly among the high rolling, revenue-generating stars of the OR, saw it as an opportunity to bring their aggressions to bear on yet another member of administration, particularly on a young, inexperienced medical director with little positional power and only a modicum of personal power, which might well be dribbled away after a brief honeymoon period.

My first foray into management was not met with applause from the troops, but the position attracted me. The promised tedium of meetings offered the possibility for creating change. Perhaps, as Mitch Rabkin, MD, then President of Beth-Israel Medical Center in Boston, said to me years later, "All the patients are mine, and I feel responsible for all of them. I work for all of them." Besides, it looked like fun.

In the late 1970s, hospital vice-presidents for medical affairs (VPMAs) were still somewhat of a novelty. The membership of the (then) American Academy of Medical Directors numbered fewer than 200, and more than a few of that meager number saw the position as a novel carriage to retirement rather than as the launching pad for the new career that it has become today.

In those first years, meetings, often poorly planned and poorly managed, became my main means of work; groups of people replaced the lone patient and his or her parents. The change was palpable. The excitement of being "in on the ground floor" frequently gave way to the tedium of the mundane and a clinician's frustration that answers were slow in coming and that change was slow to happen.

A few clinicians were only too happy to remind me of these impediments during my frequent visits to the physicians' lounge. "No, it's not in the budget." "I'll talk to them." "Our staffing is great in spite of what you may feel." These and others like them became my standard replies. The traditional spheres of influence and responsibilities of VPMAs and medical directors (medical affairs, graduate education, medical library, quality assurance, and continuing medical education) were not on the cutting edge of administrative decision-making and strategy. They often did not command budget and staffing resources needed to effect change.

It seemed to me that the path to greater effectiveness was through operating rather than staff departments. I hoped to "paint with a broader brush." I had a strong mentor, and the environment encouraged physician involvement. The other managers were also willing to work within that culture. Thus, I became managerially responsible for all of the clinical departments, working closely with their physician leadership and their management directors. This alliance proved to be beneficial for the department chairs, who felt they now had an even stronger voice in management decisions.

Those early years of line responsibility for performance, people, budget, and outcomes not only proved to be a critical learning experience for me, but also enabled me to gain the credibility to move to a top management position a few years later. Indeed, the opportunity to manage both the medicine and the money was a critical step in my career development.

Reorganization of health care organizations, particularly hospitals, became fashionable in the early eighties as one-stop-shopping, the corporate model, mergers, and joint ventures became the new sirens of organizational design strategy. Like corporate America, the health care industry was re-inventing itself. In the resulting chaos came opportunity, and I became the executive vice president and chief operating officer of the enterprise, now responsible for all hospital and medical group operating departments. It was a BIG job, and I felt I was ready. It was a glorious time. We were on the move, and I was an integral part of the excitement. The medical staff was supportive and played a key part in selecting my successor as VPMA.

But big jobs create big headaches; the frustrations and anxiety of the office began to squeeze some of the zest from the day…and night. As clinical decision makers, physicians are accustomed to an almost immediate response: the newborn turns from blue to pink after the procedure, a fracture is repaired, the heart patient returns to home and work. The rewards of the profession are immediate; gratification in successfully managing a "difficult case" warms the spirit and the intellect. The patient and me: one on one.

The process of management frequently takes much longer and nearly always depends on the participation of many others. Rewards for a budget well done, a project well managed, a marketing campaign successfully orchestrated are most often delayed, sometimes by years. That's a challenge. In my counseling of physician executives beginning careers in management, the delay of processes and their own impatience have been their greatest sources of frustration. Many in new positions of management seem to be Type A personalities frustrated by driving Type B buses. Or they feel like NASCAR drivers in a tractor pull.

These inner challenges were significant and, at times, disquieting. Learning new approaches, styles, and methods was both fun and frustrating, but none of it hurt. However, firing a co-worker, particularly one who has helped the organization progress and prosper, can be gut-wrenching. Organizations lose people for a variety of reasons. Some move on for better career opportunities, for family reasons, or for other reasons over which you have no control. A few simply sense that it's time to move on. Old baggage has piled up; there have been too many shortfalls and slips;

performance has been marginal. You get the letter of resignation, give a sigh of relief, and start the search for a replacement.

The tough departures are those who don't want to go, who don't see their shortfalls, or whose skills and talents no longer meet organizational needs. The decision to "fire" is tough. When it becomes easy, it's your turn to move on.

In preparing background material for a course I have taught called "Change and Innovation," I surveyed dozens of physician executives, particularly CEOs, asking them for the hardest action they have ever had to take as an executive. The responses have been almost uniform: because they are trained to heal not to hurt, firing people was the most challenging and personally stressful task. As clinicians our accountability is primarily to the patient, to the profession. As executives that responsibility and accountability are largely to an organization of people, an institution with its own mission and purpose.

There were other challenges—disciplining physicians, rage management, decisions driven by greed, and tremendous resistance to change are also high on my list of dissatisfiers. They challenged my abilities and patience and took me out of my comfort zone. I took a course about "whole brain" thinking that described the characteristics of "left brain" and "right brain" dominant people. The take-away lesson was that we each possess different talents and that none of us possess them all. I learned more about my talent and skill list and about my shortfalls. Performance evaluations, something virtually unknown to clinicians, became a source of benefit to me, because peers and board members proved to have insights I did not. As a result we carefully and deliberately built teams of diverse people with different skill sets. Thankfully, many were "left brainers" whose attention to detail and sequence complemented the "big picture" right brain strategy I found easier to see. The budget became a strategic weapon only because of the detailers, the operating people, the tacticians, and the folks who make it happen. They became the core strength of the enterprise and a great legacy for my successor. They saved my career as chief operating officer.

Like so many others in the field, we, too, came down with a near fatal case of merger mania in the late eighties and nineties. Corporate America was doing it, consolidating into behemoths that promised miracles of efficiency and effectiveness. Why couldn't health care, America's largest single business, learn these lessons? It was change at its best and at its worst!

Our first trek into this wilderness was squashed by the U.S. Department of Justice, which argued that we might not be as altruistic as we promised and that both clout and cost were the only things likely to increase. The

Third Circuit Court of Appeals held the same view, and the consolidation crashed.

Once again change, if not chaos, created opportunity. I became President and CEO of the health system. It was my fifteenth year with the organization. My longevity, familiarity, and local success eliminated the need for a search. I recall a recruiter saying much earlier in my career that I should move on every few years, taking on new challenges and rounding out my resume in order to become a viable candidate for CEO positions. Maybe. I had been afforded personal growth from within the organization and had established a track record there, including a list of not-so-successful endeavors I was allowed to repair. I knew the culture. So I told him that I found that it's often harder to stay in one place and have to face and fix the mistakes you've made. I think moving on is second to staying and growing responsibility from within if possible.

The ravages of corporate America during 2002 catalyzed a lot of second thoughts about the processes of the for-profit world, particularly the selection of CEOs. The *New York Times* reports[2] that "corporations have it all wrong." Corporate America goes outside for executive talent as "regular as rain," but the results have been far short of expectations. Turnover is high, successors at troubled companies don't necessarily do better that their predecessors. Indeed, hiring outsiders is "negatively correlated with dramatic improvements," and as a result more companies seem willing to invest time and money to develop executive leadership from within. While comparisons between health care management and the Wall Streeters who make the news is hazardous, the observation nevertheless bears some examination. Short of performance disasters, a radical shift in strategy, a scandal, or credibility gap, more corporations may well do better from internal development and promotion.

Being CEO was different from anything I had previously experienced. The initial days in office were joyous. I had the chance to put it all together in ways that were not possible earlier. The health system became my enterprise to guide, to lead, and to be responsible for. I had been in the organization for 15 years, and its future success became quite personal.

That was in the early 1990s, and it still feels good to have been given that opportunity. However, the loneliness of responsibility and leadership cannot be easily dismissed. The accountability that is at once invigorating would also prove to be confining and frustrating. I found it harder, though not impossible, to stay close to the spirit of the organization's people. Clean answers and candor became a little more difficult to get from some who were awed by the office. Certainly, my peer network was responsive and empathetic, frequently offering support, insight, and perspective.

Despite a collaborative process and a responsive Board of Directors, the aloneness of decision making, responsibility, and accountability was with me 24 hours a day, 7 days a week. All decisions, including those made by others, became mine. During times of uncertainty or ambiguity, the counsel of board members was particularly helpful. Often I assembled the "kitchen cabinet," a short list of the more experienced and wiser board members, to test ideas, express concerns, and ask for guidance outside of the boardroom. Their advice also provided insight on how best to develop the board and use its individual and collective talents. These experienced guides and coaches proved to be important anchors in a chaotic industry.

Organizations display many examples of chaotics at work. They are complex, dynamic, inter-connected, blends of people often pulling in many directions and motivated by different needs. What then allows organizations to be successful in such potential turbulence? More to the point, what do successful leaders do that prevents these dynamic and biotic enterprises from simply coming apart under centrifugal force? Why do people go to work, extend themselves, work the extra shifts, tolerate the challenges? I have been in the 24 x 7 business for three decades, and have been in awe of those who solve its staffing challenges and have marveled at technicians and nurses who agree to take the extra shift; care for the extra patient. How does," you couldn't pay me enough" morph into running the extra mile? I think you'll find in successful business cultures a force that counterbalances chaos, a kind of organizational glue, and that glue is called meaning. Effective leaders bring meaning to the efforts of their followers. "I will follow you," they might say, "if what you do and what you stand for brings me purpose, an appreciation, and a feeling that it and I are valuable". Successful leaders align their words, deeds, actions, rewards, pictures, to give meaning beyond the immediate. Successful leaders have followers because followers want to be where the leader wants to go.

President Dwight Eisenhower said it well. "Leadership is the art of getting someone else to do something you want done because he wants to do it." Charles Dwyer, former Professor of Business at the Wharton School, said it most instructively, "Don't expect someone to behave in a way that satisfies your values unless it also satisfies their values."

The use of "mini-boards," advisory committees, and internal consultants for guiding projects was quite helpful in searching for common values and expectations. Savvy individuals, knowledgeable but not directly in the operating line of responsibility, can provide valuable insight into the numerous obstacles, false starts, and group politics that typically "dog" the management of change. In addition, organizations often have a small group of "early adopters," those more willing to embrace change, to follow a lead, to experiment with the new. These individuals can be an crucial part of any change process or quality improvement team. Most others, you should expect, will be more resistant; some simply dig in their heels for the duration, and a few may become downright subversive. For those resisting, the greater the change to their own work patterns and daily habits, the more threatening to their value systems (including money), the greater the obstacles they are likely to create. It is no surprise, therefore, that major changes to the landscape, like mergers, the computerized office record, physician order entry, and new facilities can create major challenges for the executive leading the process.

I have found a few strategies for change to be particularly effective: identify the stakeholders and over-communicate early; use pilots that can be modified by input from the stakeholders, and include a broad cast of the early adopters. Once involved, these progressives can serve as role models for their peers. I'm reminded of our efforts to install a bedside computer system on a surgical floor. Resistance melted when one of the more conservative physicians was persuaded by his office nurse to give it a try. Once seen at the keyboard by others, he achieved icon status, and the installation proceeded almost uneventfully.

We were involved in merger mania two more times while I was CEO. The promises of cost management, if not control, economies of scale, and bargaining clout sang what could be realized through merger, loudly. A chorus of consultants added to the score. Even the Justice Department smiled this time. But, as with so many other attempts to change and to control costs, the strategy came up short both times. Both attempts were efforts to move an organization that was unwilling to change its historically successful ways.

Those years in pursuit of merger were undoubtedly the most stressful ones in my career. I paced the backyard at 2 a.m., looking for answers in the stars, hoping to have asked the right questions. Merger is perhaps the most disruptive of strategies: a curious and challenging alchemy of opinion, fact, community, physician expectations and demands, politics, personal agendas, secret meetings, and public pronouncements. The potential benefits were widely extolled: cost reduction, efficiency of capital and operations, bargaining and purchasing leverage, and better use of soon-to-be underutilized facilities. Prowess at recruiting and the possibilities of expanded medical education programs were also touted. For those whose jobs and culture survive the marriage, there are bigger challenges, broader responsibilities, and higher pay.

But the promises come only with great change to working relationships and habits; organizational values and cultures are threatened; resistance is common, particularly in that phase of realistic doubt that springs from the discoveries of due diligence. The expectation of the merging parties can be quite divergent. Representation on the new governing body, role and authority of department chairmen and managers, location of programs, centralization of authority, and religion proved to be major challenges. Culture, i.e. "what we value and how we do things around here," is part of the glue that holds many complex organizations together. Challenges to that culture proved overwhelming. We decided not to proceed and moved on.

In retrospect, it is interesting to see that merger mania has subsided, several well-publicized marriages of national fame have ended in divorce, and the promised savings and efficiencies have proven difficult to achieve.

It took several years to really learn the CEO job; to decide what was to be done; to shift from the immediacy of operations to the futurism of strategy, mission, and goals; to develop a direction. I saw five critical goals:

- Develop and implement a strategy for fulfilling our mission.
- Develop people.
- Develop systems of information management.
- Create a culture focused on quality and its measurement.
- Create a strategy and agenda for change.

In the final analysis, we are in the people business. The challenge is to make clear what is expected of ourselves and staff, to provide the tools necessary for motivated people to do their work, and to put them in a place where they can maximize their inherent talents. We relied heavily on the group process and on quality improvement teams. It became impossible to over-communicate—to "over-involve." Meaningful involvement meant construction of a unique career development ladder for every individual. Over time, the organization developed a multi-cultural, multi-talented, whole brain environment. And it served our mission well.

Among our most meaningful decisions were those that directly touched the community outside our health care missions. Encouragement of employees to be involved in community affairs, recognition and compensation for certain levels of involvement, sponsorships of school programs, and the re-development of our own neighborhood are part of our corporate responsibility, part of the obligation incurred through our tax exemption. With the help of Habitat for Humanity and our city's government, we relocated streets, rehabilitated homes, built houses for those otherwise left behind, built a children's playground, and subsidized housing. Community accountability and outreach, stretching beyond what is "given at the office," is part of the people business we're in and among the most rewarding of CEO initiatives. It's part of leading beyond the bottom line.

As retired CEO and current board Chairman, I read the trade magazines with a little more leisure. There's more time to think, ask, and ponder. I wonder how often mergers have delivered on their promises. How often have prices stabilized after a merger, let alone declined as hoped. I wonder how long we can continue to manage a trillion dollar industry with paper records, note cards, and Post-Its? While the technology that has saved my life on more than one occasion continues to improve, if not astound, the infrastructure upon which it is delivered is fatally flawed. How can the next generation of leaders bring about reform, more standardized protocols, and universal coverage and access? Once again the field has reversed direction, undoing consolidation, practice acquisitions, insurance company creations, and single-source strategies that dominated the early '90s. What can we learn from this?

As Chairman, I now see our system from another aspect, a far different view than I saw as a young physician. As clinician the hospital was my employer and my "workshop," the place to take my patients, the source of technology and staffing. "Administration" was symbolized by the head nurse, and the blurred suits of higher management who maneuvered somewhere unseen in the background or in the board room. I didn't know how it all worked or why it worked. I didn't understand the glue that holds all the organizational chaos together: the hospital's mission to heal and the staff's knowledge that its work is important.

It's now a unique privilege to observe the entire organization from a background of both operations and strategy, to watch the efforts of so many years blossom in new people and successor teams, to watch the ground change with new facilities and better programs. It is hard to break the habit of work, to leave the challenges to the next order of talent, to try and become a wise old coach and seer. But the reward of it all has been intense, lasting, refreshing, and humbling. Unmet challenges remain.

As a patient I have seen the system from yet a fourth perspective. As the victim of a heart attack years ago, I was blessed by being in a country where access to first-rate acute care is expected and common. Magnificent technology, talent, medications, and guidance produced a wonderful and sustainable result in hours to days. Sometime later, I became a survivor of cancer, a horrible burden we're all fighting to turn into a chronic disease. Travels through that part of our endeavors quickly expose some of the weaknesses of an acute care, response-driven "system." I found a non-system, a collage of busy health components and cottage industries, often disconnected from the greater demands of chronic recurrent disease. If ever there was a role for the physician executive, I believe it is here. The collision of office practice, surgicenter, hospital, pharmacy, technology, prevention, information systems, and money is a din of dis-coordination. Here is fertile ground for rebuilding a flawed infrastructure. Here, I believe, are the career options of tomorrow.

Mother no longer cries about my choice, and most clinicians that I know no longer feel that physician executives have been lost to the other side of suits and meetings. The field has blossomed, but challenges to prove our worth remain. Years ago, when beginning in this field and feeling particularly threatened by one of our clinical barracudas, I sought some common ground and understanding. I said, "You seem to feel that I'm no longer a doctor standing here, now that I've joined 'them.'" He replied, "No, you don't understand. You're no longer a clinician, but you'll always be a doctor. Good luck."

References

1.   Naisbitt, J. *Megatrends: Ten New Directions Transforming Our Lives*. New York, N.Y.: Warner Books, 1982.

2.   Gabor, A. "Challenging a Corporate Addiction to Outsiders." *New York Times*, Nov. 17, 2002, Section 3, p. 4.

Robert B. Klint, MD, MHA, FACPE, was chairman of the board of SwedishAmerican Health System in Rockford, Ill. when this chapter was written. He previously served as president and CEO. SwedishAmerican comprises a major acute care hospital, a network of primary care and multispecialty clinics, home health care branches and an ambulatory surgery facility. Dr. Klint succombed to colon cancer in 2004 after a three-year fight.

Chapter 2

Key Management Skills for the Physician Executive

by Leland R. Kaiser, PhD

This chapter is written for you, a physician executive employed in a modern health care organization. The chapter will help you reconceptualize your job and identify some of the key management skills you must master to be successful. The skills I describe are drawn from the current management literature and from my experience in working with physician executives. A bibliography is attached for further study.

Role of the Physician Executive

You are an interface professional. You work on the interface between the disciplines of medicine and management. Most of the problems in our contemporary health care system fall on this interface. A good example of an interface problem is the trade-off between cost and quality of medical care. This trade-off requires that both a medical and a management decision be made for each patient. You are qualified to make such decisions because you have expertise in both arenas and can simultaneously protect the patient's and the organization's welfare.

Your role and function will vary with the needs and interests of your employer. As a result of the wide range of job functions that physician executives perform, there is no uniform job description. In each new position, you must negotiate your role and function with your employer. You must match your interests and abilities to the job that needs to be done.

Advocating for both the patient and the organization places the physician executive in a value conflict situation. What is best for the patient is not always best for the organization. What is best for the organization is not always best for the community. What is best for the community is not always best for the federal government. A manager always faces conflicts of interest. The physician has the luxury of focusing only upon the needs of patients. You must take into account the interests of all the parties involved. Learning to think like a manager as well as a physician is one of your greatest challenges. You have mixed accountability, and often what makes one party happy with you will make another party angry with you. Good managers try to plan "win-win" games, but it is not always possible to do this in the real world of the physician executive.

Any manager is expected to promote the institution's philosophy and uphold its goals. You must be a team player and accept your role as a co-creator of your organization. You must be concerned not only with medical management problems, but also with the general welfare of your organization. This requires that you identify with organizational interests and problems that transcend your day-to-day functioning as a medical care administrator.

An alert physician executive will keep his or her organization well informed concerning new developments in medicine and patient care. This requires careful monitoring of the literature and attendance at medical meetings. You are expected to be an expert source for medical management, and other organizational managers will depend on your advice and direction.

The physician executive is expected to set the standard of excellence for physicians in the organization. You must play a leadership role in quality assurance and risk management. The medical staff should view you first as a doctor, then as a manager. The management team, by contrast, will view you first as a manager, then as a doctor. Because you live in both camps, from time to time you must engage in a little fancy footwork, convincing both doctors and managers that you are representing their respective interests.

Some physician executives continue to see patients; others do not. There is no simple rule to follow in this matter. The important thing is that you maintain clinical credibility with the other physicians in your organization. That is hard to do if you no longer see patients. Yet even if you continue to see patients, it will be difficult for you to maintain medical competence on a part-time practice basis and even harder to find enough hours in the day to also practice management. Most physician executives gradually move toward full-time management because of these twin pressures. Some physician executives want to keep a foot in both camps because they are not yet fully committed to the management role and want to keep their bases covered just in case they decide to return to full-time practice.

As a physician executive, you will be subjected to many organizational challenges and stresses. Being an interface professional is not easy work. Potential stresses include:

- The time and effort it takes to stay current in two disciplines.
- Dual identity as both a physician and a manager (this can lead to an identity conflict or a feeling you are neither).
- Lack of role clarity in your organization.
- Less hands-on satisfaction than you had as a pure clinician.
- Trying to quickly learn the required new management skills.
- Excessive work loads.
- Being in the middle between the medical staff and management (conflict).
- Having few professional peers to relate to (loneliness).

If you are successful in your organizational role, you will mediate, translate, integrate, and absorb shock. These situations are stress generating, and you must develop some good stress management skills if you hope to remain healthy in the job.

Of course, there are many benefits that go along with this exciting new profession:

- Exploration of a new career.
- Variety and change.
- Identification with an organization (security and protection).
- Exercise of power and control.
- The challenge of mastering a new body of knowledge.

The pluses outweigh the minuses, but you must factor them both into the equation of overall job satisfaction. Learning to think like a manager represents one of the biggest challenges you will face. Characteristics of the mindset of a manager include:

- Seeing the big picture.
- Adopting organizational values and standards.
- Engaging in objective analytical thinking.
- Acting in the face of uncertainty.
- Enjoying complexity.
- Developing goals and objectives.
- Translating goals and objectives into action plans.

- Measuring organizational effectiveness.
- Developing a distinctive style of leadership.
- Assessing organizational effectiveness.

Though these skills are not antithetical to those of a physician, they are not usually well developed as a result of medical school education or clinical practice. Some physicians have a natural bent for management and have picked up some of the necessary skills. For other physicians, thinking like a manager is something that must be learned and practiced before proficiency is developed.

A physician gets direct positive reinforcement from patients. The physician is recognized and appreciated for what he or she does for them. A manager must depend upon vicarious reinforcement. He or she succeeds only through the efforts of others. Reward is second-hand at best. Often, good management goes unnoticed, and all you will receive are a lot of complaints if something goes wrong. People are unconscious of good management and are therefore unlikely to notice it when it occurs. If you want to feel good about yourself, you may have to pat yourself on the back for a job well done. Some physician executives miss the "good old days" when they were really appreciated by their patients.

It is important for the physician executive to develop a strong working relationship with the nursing manager. Both are clinician executives and working together can constitute a powerful force for change in the organization. After all, who can successfully oppose all the doctors and nurses in the organization? The nursing manager is working on the interface between nursing and management and must have many of the same skills and interests as the physician executive. They are major allies and should view each other as equals in the process of planning and delivering patient care.

Innovation is an important role for the physician executive. He or she should stimulate creative thinking in the organization and be a major force for new product development. Most physicians are trained to think conservatively, and innovation is often outside their interest and experience in providing patient care. An innovator is a risk taker and must be willing to make many mistakes in the process of developing successful business ventures. Although by temperament some physicians are entrepreneurs, few physicians have had experience stimulating innovation in organizational settings. Physician executives working in hospitals may wish to set aside some beds on a special research and development unit where new approaches to patient care can be tested and evaluated for cost, quality, and patient satisfaction. In some instances, the unit becomes a strategy for total organizational change as innovations developed there are accepted throughout the hospital by other caregivers. Patient-focused care is a good research and development project if the hospital has not already incorporated it into its philosophy and practice.

Managers spend more time communicating than engaging in any other management behavior. A primary role of the physician executive is to serve as a communication link between the medical staff and management. He or she must properly represent the perceptions of each to the other. Written and verbal communication, dyads, small groups, large groups, and public speaking all fall within his or her purview. The physician executive who is not an effective communicator might benefit from some further training in the communications department of a local college or university.

Ultimately, as the new kid on the block, you must make your own way in the organization. Your position as a physician executive will be what you make it. Your profession is new enough that health care organizations do not have a lot of preconceived notions about what you should do. You do not have to cut through a lot of history. You do have to become an architect of your future in the organization. If you are creative and quick to see how you can contribute, you will write your own ticket. If you wait to be asked, you may wait for a long time.

A major challenge may be resisting the avalanche of problems that beset you when you first arrive in the organization. We all have a tendency to react to whatever is demanding our attention. We have an inclination to do whatever we enjoy doing and are good at, whether or not it needs to be done. Discrimination is an important managerial skill. You must constantly ask yourself, "What most needs to be done in this organization at this time?" If you do not plan your work and your day, you will be swept away by trivia and will never have time to do the really important things. Your time is your most precious resource—learn to guard it carefully. There are too many good things to do and too few that will make any long-term difference for either your organization or your patients. Stand back and get perspective. Ask yourself, "Why am I doing this?"

Becoming a Professional Manager

You will achieve success by doing what you do best. Where you are the weakest, you will fail. The effective manager concentrates on what he does well and hires other people to do what he does poorly. Be sure to hire associates who are unlike you and do not share your weaknesses. Much of your career success depends on the match between who you are and where you are. Much also depends on your skill in surrounding yourself with competent subordinates. How well do you fit your current organizational space?

What do you need from your organization to really do the job? If you designed the ideal job space for yourself, how would it look? A manager that is a failure in one organizational setting is often a success in another organization. Everything depends on fit. If the organization does not fit you—you are a misfit. You need a good fit between your personal profile and the map of your organizational environment. Here, self-knowledge is all important.

Where is your organization in its life cycle? Organizations, like people, have life cycles. Organizations are born, grow rapidly, reach maturity, and decline. It is more fun to manage an organization in its period of rapid growth than its decline. Many physician executives are being hired by relatively new health care organizations. This adds an element of excitement and optimism to the position. The downside is that many of these organizations are unstable, economically risky, and subject to disappearance. You may be forced to trade the security of maturity for the excitement of youth. Managing an organization in decline is a no-win situation. Remember, as a manager, your destiny is tied to the destiny of your organization. It pays to be a little choosy and not necessarily pick the job with the highest salary and greatest fringe benefits. It may not be around long enough for you to collect either.

Are your organization's values consistent with your values? Values are the lowest common denominator of action both in people and in organizations. You cannot be an effective manager if you do not agree with what your organization is doing. The best management is management by value. What are the corporate values of your organization? What are your personal and professional values as a physician executive? Are both sets of values consistent? If not, what do you need to do? Some organizations do not have a very clear sense of their values and need to go through a value clarification process.

Are you overtrained for your job? A professional manager feels best when he or she is challenged but not overwhelmed. Boredom is as difficult to live with as too much excitement. What is your optimal stimulus level as a manager? Do you feel a sense of accomplishment in your job and an opportunity to bring your full range of abilities into action?

Are you being adequately compensated for what you do? A physician executive should enjoy a high standard of living and a full return on the tremendous investment made in his or her career. You should compare your salary and benefits with other physician executives in comparable jobs. You may experience a decrease in income when you switch from fee-for-service, solo practice to an organizational salary. However, your expenses are less, you enjoy more free time, and the security is greater. As with everything in life, becoming a physician executive is a trade-off.

Did anyone precede you in your position? If so, you will inherit some organizational expectations created by the previous holder of your office. These may be good, bad, or, more likely, a mix. Talk to other people and try to recreate a picture of the world before you arrived. Decide what was right and wrong with that world and announce to the organization any needed changes you will be making. If you are going to make changes, the burden of proof is upon you.

Organizations always resist change. You may experience some of this resistance as you try to cut a new groove for your position. It also helps to know the history of your organization. Organizations are where they have been. Who were the founders? What were the major milestones in the development of the organization? By knowing the traditions and symbols of the organization, you enter its mythology and stand the best chance of helping in the transformation of the myth as the organization prepares to move into the future. The myth of the organization is its tap root and should always be taken seriously. Kill the tap root and the organization dies. Set yourself against the traditions of the organization and you will surely lose.

As a professional manager, you must build your knowledge base and remain open to new ideas. Every month you should peruse the leading management journals and read several of the best books on management. As we enter the turbulent information age in health care, new age managers will be practicing management by idea. Organizations that survive this "white water" period will be the "better idea" organizations. You will never be a better manager than your knowledge base permits. What you cannot think about, you cannot manage. There are few rules in management and little memory work. Management is primarily conceptual. A good manager is not a technician. He or she is a well-read thinker.

Because the role of physician executive is filled with ambiguity, it is important for you to project a strong self-concept. You must tell other people who you are and what you do. In some cases it is important to tell the organization what you do not do. It is tempting for an organization to load you up with things you should not be doing. You should be doing only what a person with your experience and dual training is qualified to do. If you are performing lower level tasks, the organization is wasting money and losing the unique contribution only you can make.

There are three big questions that any manager asks:

- What should I be doing (values)?
- How can I do that (knowledge)?
- Who can do it (power)?

This is the equilateral triangle of management. A physician executive must manage values, knowledge, and power. Unless you are willing to become a power broker, your values and knowledge will not come to fruition. Organizations are political creatures. Management decisions are often made on political grounds and fly in the face of both analysis and intellect. You must seek power in order to make a difference in your organization. You can only receive power from those who have power to bestow. For this reason, your relationship to the CEO and the board is critical. Without the support of those higher up in the power structure, you will not be effective and you will end up frustrated—able to see but not able to do.

Any professional manager depends on a network of colleagues to provide support and information. The physician executive needs such a reference group to avoid professional isolation. Begin cultivating professional contacts with other physician executives if you have not already done so. Stay in touch by phone and letter and arrange to meet at national and regional meetings of your professional societies.

Relationship with the Chief Executive Officer

Be certain the CEO supports you and your function in the organization. Work with the CEO to develop a clear job description and a location on the organizational chart that gives you a direct reporting line to the CEO. Obtain a commitment from the CEO for adequate budgetary and staff support. You should also request a three- to five-year employment contract after the first year or two of employment.

Work with the CEO to define your major goals and objectives for the fiscal year. Tie these goals to your budget and to your performance review. Make sure the CEO and you agree on organizational priorities and on your allocations of time and effort. Keep the CEO informed concerning your progress on goal achievement. If any unexpected events intrude on your projected work program, discuss them with the CEO and have him or her sign off on any changes in priorities. Your value to the CEO will depend primarily on the extent to which you keep your assigned organizational areas problem-free (do your job) and the degree to which you assist the CEO with his or her own perplexities (help the CEO with his or her job). It will pay you to spend some time every week worrying about the CEO's problems and suggesting possible solutions. Worry about what the boss is worried about, and you won't have to worry about the boss.

Request frequent feedback from the CEO and give the CEO frequent feedback. The most important part of your job is communication. If you want to enjoy a long and happy life in your organization, demonstrate consistent loyalty to the CEO and volunteer for jobs the CEO needs to have accomplished. Before long he or she will depend on your input every week.

Relationship to the Management Team

To be effective over the long haul, you must build a high level of trust with other members of the management team. Be certain that team members understand your role and function. Be certain they are satisfied with your performance. Always be prepared for organizational meetings and perform well in them. Performance in meetings is a major criterion used to evaluate any manager. Most of the work of an organization is done in meetings. From time to time, you will tire of meetings. Resist the temptation to bad mouth meetings. You will only lose ground with this or any other occasion of organizational criticism. Carry your share of the work load and always document your accomplishments with other team members. Encourage divergent opinions from the group, but avoid adversarial relationships with any team members. Aim for consensus decision making.

It is important for you to be available and approachable. Display company manners. Give frequent praise. Be a good listener. You need to be highly visible in the organization and to practice management by walking around.

Become a student of the organization's written policies and procedures. Play by the rules. If a rule needs to be changed, volunteer to study the rule and suggest a new policy better adapted to the changing health care environment. You win points on any management team by being predictable, open, fair, and loyal in your dealings with all team members. The time may come when your job tenure is decided by your team members. Avoid making enemies at any level of the organization. Remember, it takes a lot more effort to fight a war than to maintain the peace.

Because many changes are taking place on the interface between medicine and management, you should conduct frequent briefing meetings for team members. Organizations do not like surprises, and it is your job to see that none occur in your assigned areas. If you have important fears or doubts about what is happening in patient care, share your feelings with the group.

Relationship with the Medical Staff

One of your most important functions is maintaining positive relationships with other physicians. In hospitals and clinics, this usually takes the form of your interactions with the organized medical staff. Some physician executives believe the medical staff cannot be organized, and that simple fact alone is the root of most of their problems. It is not easy to organize doctors, yet that is your job.

Your transactions with doctors can take many forms. You may be involved in recruiting doctors for your organization. You may call on physicians in their private offices, offer practice management consultation, and act as a liaison to the hospital. Office-based physicians often welcome help with marketing and sale of their services. If the doctors do well, the hospital should also prosper. It is a "win-win" game. Often, physician executives develop orientation programs for new doctors joining the staff. The orientation program provides an excellent opportunity for you to explain the institution's culture and make organizational expectations clear to new physicians.

An important part of your role is to mobilize physician commitment to your organization's services. You may meet this challenge by initiating a medical staff development program that encourages physician input in organizational decision making and makes doctors part of the family. If you can develop a core leadership group as a result of your medical staff development program, you will find your job as a change agent much easier.

By providing financial and clinical outcome data to physicians, you can improve their performance. Prompt feedback motivates doctors to do a better job. If possible, medical education should be geared to problems documented in the performance reviews. As a physician executive, you must monitor physician practice patterns and estimate their impact on quality and cost outcomes. Sometimes it is a simple matter of keeping physician skills up to date. It may, however, come to dealing with the impaired physician or the physician who must be given reduced privileges. You will have to discipline physicians who are bad actors and coach failing physicians. In matters of discipline, you will work closely with the hospital attorney to protect the rights of all parties involved.

As a physician executive, you must set up an accountability framework for physicians and enforce the ethical and legal standards of your organization and your profession. This is never a pleasant task for a manager, but it is one that must be done. In these matters, the buck stops at your desk.

Part of your role as a physician executive is to teach other physicians to think like managers. You may need to hold some special educational sessions to explain all of the changes coming down the road that will affect doctors and hospitals. Physicians need help in learning to manage reimbursement and admission policies. Payer mix is an important variable in determining the hospital's economic survival. The physician is the major resource allocator in health care organizations and needs to understand his or her economic impact on the organization.

An important future role for physician executives will be developing new corporate structures that bring doctors and hospitals together as financial partners. No longer can doctors and hospitals compete with one another or choose to go their separate ways. They will hang together or hang separately. Physician/hospital organizations, IPAs, hospital-based group practices, integrated regional health care networks, primary care networks, hospital/community HMOs, direct contracting, and capitated managed care are only a few of the new corporate forms that may be needed in the reform and postreform periods of American health care. There is ample opportunity and incentive for creative experimentation by all health provider organizations.

Future health care will be dominated by computers and information networks. You need to view information systems as the new wave of medicine and management. How familiar are you with computers? Do you have hands-on skills? Now is a good time to begin experimenting with the new hardware and software being developed for physicians and hospitals. Does your hospital provide computerized literature searches for your physicians? Do you have a special shelf in you medical library devoted to books on computers and medicine? Are you using computers to help you with critical paths, clinical outcome measurements, and order entry?

Product line management is still a promising way to plan and deliver health care in multispecialty group practices and hospitals. A production team composed of doctors, nurses, and other personnel plans the products for each specialty area in medicine. Market segments, packaging, distribution channels, volume, profit margins, and quality standards are determined for each specialty each year. Product performance is measured against production targets, and exceptions are noted and corrected. As a product manager, you can decide to position your products for cost, quality, service, or convenience. If you can position for all four, so much the better.

Service is becoming an important emphasis in health care. As a physician executive, you should help develop a customer service strategy for your institution. With extensive competitive bidding for contracts, cost and quality differentials will even out among providers and the emphasis will be on the user interface. Do you provide a good experience for the patient and family?

The dispirited physician is a phenomenon of our times. Many doctors are discouraged and have decided to leave the clinical practice of medicine. Early retirements and career changes are common. Part of your job is to maintain physician esprit de corps and do what you can to add hope and help to disheartened doctors who feel they have been betrayed by society.

Competition among medical facilities will continue to increase until collaboration is finally recognized as the strategy of choice for health care in the United States. You must develop an effective plan for monitoring the competition and meeting it in the marketplace. What is your organization's distinctive competence? Can you develop centers of excellence? Where do you have the greatest depth in your medical and nursing staffs? Can you protect and extend your primary care base? Can you install more effective cost controls? Can you improve channels of distribution? How will the growth of managed care affect your profit margins? Are you ready for new methods of physician reimbursement? Does your governing board recognize the changing medical market?

An important role you have with the medical staff is that of change agent. You are paid to help doctors change the way they think. Each year, you should take a carefully selected group of doctors and managers on site visits to view innovative solutions to problems experienced in your institution. One site visit will change more physicians' minds than years of admonition and pleading. This means that you must maintain a list of innovation sites. This can be done by a careful search of the literature and by calling on your professional network of physician executives.

A routine but important job of the hospital-based physician executive is liaison with designated clinical, managerial, and governance committees. When appropriate, the physician executive should attempt to improve the functioning of these committees and their relationships with each other. If the hospital takes regular physician and nurse polls, the physician executive should be involved in the polling and the interpretation of results.

Joint ventures, mergers, consolidations, and coalitions, still represent important new arenas for physician executive involvement. These are complex organizational arrangements, and you should approach them with caution. A good business plan will avert many potential disasters. You should be able to read, understand, and evaluate business plans for any proposed organizational relationship. Consultants can help you in this area. Do not hesitate to use them. In the future, medical staffs will be more involved in these decisions. There will also be increased pluralism in all health provider organizations. Although the movement will be toward larger organizations, some doctors will continue as solo practitioners.

Other physicians will join large multispecialty groups and regional integrated corporations that promise greater power and financial return.

Relationship with the Community

The mission of a medical care system is to improve the health status of the population it serves. Because the provision of disease care is only one element in the improvement of overall community health status, many physician executives will be extensively involved in community health outreach programs with schools, churches, business and industry, recreation departments, public health, welfare, housing, criminal justice, and transportation. The hospital will become a community health design center and an institution "without walls." Primary care will be decentralized to the neighborhood level. Attempts will be made to judge effectiveness of area medical care providers by measurable improvement in community health status. As medicine becomes population-based, accountability of doctors and hospitals can be determined and measured. Creating healthier communities is a new frontier for physician executives.

Relationship with Federal, State, and Local Government

A logical career progression for physicians is from clinician to physician executive to health policy analyst. Most of the health legislation in the United States is drafted by legislative aides who have never treated a patient or spent time managing a health care institution. That alone explains why much of our health legislation is so woefully inadequate. In the future, self-selected physician executives who have met the challenge of institutional management will go on to the policy arena. They will draw on their rich and diversified patient, organizational, and community experience to craft laws of the land. Of course, the political process in the legislatures will still operate, but it will be operating from an expert physician base.

Essential Professional Skills of the Physician Executive

As I indicated earlier, as a professional manager you will spend more time communicating than engaging in any other organizational behavior. Listening skills, personal observation skills, self-disclosure skills, and the ability to write and speak well are essential. You will communicate one-to-one, in small groups, in large groups, and on occasion before large audiences. Your ability to influence, motivate, and persuade others will determine much of your success in the organization. If you are a high-energy person, you can communicate your zest and vitality. If you are a serious, thoughtful person, you can communicate your solid grasp of problem situations. If you are a good listener, other people will seek you out to help them clarify their own thinking.

To win the confidence of your organization, you must avoid extremism. You will always be looking for the common denominator that will bring conflicting parties to resolution. You cannot afford to alienate a large part of the organization by adopting extreme positions. You are an organizational diplomat and must be able to see the validity of many points of view. Your constituents will promote conflicting ideologies and hold limiting assumptions. You must lend a friendly ear to both. You are a listening post for the organization and a mirror for those who want to see themselves through your eyes. If both liberal and conservative physicians respect you and view you as a friend, you are projecting the right image. Of course, you have your own opinions, but they should not get in the way of your managerial function as an interface professional—equally at home on either side of the fence.

A physician executive needs to be a high-energy person. On every side, you will be confronted by organizational inertia and physician passivity. Many of the battles you fight you will win because you can hold out longer than your opponents. View yourself as a spark plug. You are there to excite others to necessary action.

Your body/mind vehicle is the only tool you have as a manager. Physical and mental fitness are a precondition to organizational success. If you don't take care of yourself, you will be unable to care for the organization. Try to play a lead role in wellness programs and encourage others to conserve their health.

What theoretical perspective do you bring to your job? In my opinion, the systems perspective is the appropriate one for physician executives. You must be able to see connectedness and perceive interrelationships. Physician executives often work in complex health care organizations with multiple boards and overlapping jurisdictions. Vertical and horizontal integration, diversification, satellites, networking, joint ventures, and relationships with multiunit organizations are management realities that escape any unidimensional approach to management. You will benefit from readings in general systems theory and systems analysis.

As a physician executive, you are a change agent and must stimulate both organizational stability and organizational change. If you are prepared, you can capitalize on organizational crisis. Often, managers must wait until crisis occurs before they can motivate people to act. The good manager anticipates change and helps his organization manage it. The collective mindset of the organization is its ultimate limitation. An organization can change its future as quickly as it can change its mind. The effective physician executive is a futurist and a mind changer. New paradigm management has a quantum physics orientation. It stands in stark contrast to the Newtonian paradigm training of most physicians and managers. Quantum thinking embodies a relationship model of the universe. Newtonian thinking stresses autonomy and isolation. The physician executive must get doctors, nurses, managers, trustees, patients, and community members out of their boxes into a shared circle. The new paradigm universe is one fabric. Everything stands in relationship. Nothing stands alone. Physicians have been trained to stand alone. It is difficult for them to think organization, community, nation, or planet. Many community health and social agencies have the same problem. They think of themselves as separate and are more than willing to go to war to save their turf or budgets. As a result, most American communities are disintegrated, with huge gaps and overlaps in their services. Community health status suffers.

You need to develop your financial management skills. Everything in the organization reduces to economics. If you understand how the money flows in an organization, you understand most of the organization's dynamics. If you understand how physicians are reimbursed for their services, you can explain a lot of the variance in their practice patterns and professional behavior. You must be alert to the financial impact of all the decisions you make. Courses in cost accounting, pricing, taxes, financial management, budgeting, and investments will help you do a better job in your organization. As profit margins erode, you will become involved in downsizing, or resizing as it is often called. This may require taking beds out of service, dropping clinical services, letting employees go, and breaking relationships with managed care systems. In these instances, the required organizational decisions have both medical and managerial dimensions. Retrenchment management, as it is called, is not much fun, but it may be a necessary part of your job for the next few years.

In a rapidly changing market, your organization must decide each year what business it wants to be in. You should help your organization assess its strengths and weaknesses and reposition itself in the medical marketplace. The position your organization chooses to occupy will be translated into the type of doctors and nurses you recruit and the array of services you provide.

Effective managers create positive organizational climates and cultures of excellence. It is part of your job to clarify institutional values and convert these values into organizational behaviors. You should view yourself as a designer of the organization's culture. What kind of a medical care setting is required to ensure high-quality care and cost containment? What type of organizational climate turns physicians on and encourages physician teamwork? What does your organization really believe in, and what is it trying to accomplish? You must ask and help answer these questions.

As profit margins decline in your organization, you should be looking around for new revenue sources. An effective manager generates resources. New medical care products, new market segments, more effective marketing and sales programs, trendy packaging, optimization of existing product lines—these and other strategies will generate additional revenue. The health care field is moving toward integrated databases and data-based management. Hard facts will replace opinions as health organizations upgrade their management information systems. The physician executive needs data concerning the impact of physician practice patterns on the financial welfare of the organization. He or she can use these data to modify physician behavior. Without data, you must fly by the seat of your pants and outshout your opposition. You should update your knowledge about competing computer vendors and the information capability they provide. You should participate in the organization's decision to purchase a new computer system. Often, the information needs of the medical director are not taken into account in the buy decision. You should also use your own personal computer as a personal productivity tool. For better or worse, you will have to learn to manage with numbers.

Managed care has created a major financial problem for all health care providers. You should view yourself as a managed care consultant and help your institution select the plan that best fits its needs and financial survival. If you work for a managed care organization, you can use the same skills to design a better package for providers. Managed care is here to stay and is something you must understand. Most of the rules you have learned in fee-for-service, solo practice do not apply in this new arena.

Each year, you should review the unmet health care needs in your community and determine if they represent a desirable new market for your organization. Unmet needs may be documented and made available to the public in written reports published by other organizations in your community, such as the public health department or a local planning agency. You may have to determine the unmet needs yourself by conducting neighborhood interviews, leading consumer focus groups, or talking to the various gatekeepers in the community, such as pastors or social workers. Many communities do not offer adequate wellness programs, and there is a growing interest in such programs. Consumer interest is a key factor in your marketing effort. Who wants and is willing to pay for a product that your organization can produce? The aging population represents a growing market segment. Industrial health services is a growing niche for many health care providers. By forecasting changes in your service area, you can often spot new product opportunities.

Changes in reimbursement policy and procedure are a constant problem for all health provider organizations. The physician executive needs to examine the impact of such changes on physician behavior, organizational response, cost and quality outcomes, and organizational repositioning in the marketplace. Reimbursement is perhaps the most important dimension to understand in the business dynamics of any health care organization. Reduced reimbursement often requires cost reduction and may lead to organizational retrenchment.

As a manager, you should be alert to signs of organizational decline. This may take many forms, including an eroding community economic base, new competitors on the scene, large industries moving out of the area, increasing obsolescence of your plant and equipment, growing ineffectiveness of your board of directors, deteriorating leadership of the CEO, aging medical staff, decreasing utilization of your services, declining market share, declining net worth, increasing morale problems, a talent exodus from the organization, increasing patient care incidents, increasing litigation, renewed interest in collective bargaining, reduced quality and output, and increasing problems with third-party agencies. Organizations slowly slide into collapse if managers are not alert to the signs of decline and if they fail to engage in turnaround strategies. As a physician executive, you share responsibility for the welfare of your organization. You must alert other managers if you see signs of decline. Of course, the CEO and the board of trustees must also act. You cannot do it by yourself.

An important organizational skill for the physician executive is the ability to sell ideas and build people's enthusiasm for a better organization. You must be able to visualize a better organization and communicate that vision effectively to your fellow managers. The physician executive should be a visionary. Perhaps you should develop a think tank or futures group and get other people involved in your envisioning efforts. By creating images of possibility, the manager motivates others to excellence. Good management is high play and fun. Imagination is the key to a more abundant future for your organization.

Performance Outcomes for the Physician Executive

How do you know if you are doing your job? How will the organization measure your managerial effectiveness? Of course, your performance objectives will vary, depending on the kind of organization you are working for and the specifics of your job assignment.

The most important indicator for continued job tenure is usually how you get along with the CEO. If the CEO views you as a valuable resource and frequently consults you before making important decisions, you know you have arrived.

How popular are you with other members of the management team? Organizational satisfaction with your services is a valid indicator of your value to the organization. You can't do your job if other managers do not like and respect you. You will be evaluated on your technical expertise, interpersonal ability, and organizational participation.

Patient satisfaction is another indicator of your value to the organization. Although this is a difficult dimension to measure, you should be concerned with it. How can you increase the satisfaction of your customers? Satisfied patients tell their doctors and their friends and become repeat customers. When you manage customer satisfaction, you are managing the bottom line.

In general, the physician executive is expected to help the organization survive in the rapidly changing health care marketplace. Do you make a major contribution to the bottom line of your organization? If your organization is in the growth mode, you help it grow. If the organization is in a period of retrenchment, you help it resize. Have you been effective in your efforts to reduce costs? Whatever you do, it must be essential to the survival of the organization. If you are viewed as a luxury, your organization may not be able to afford you in a period of economic decline.

A physician executive can often help the organization expand its patient base by reaching into unserved markets. Who are potential buyers of your products who are not yet customers? A good working relationship with marketing and planning is essential in your attempt to find new patients. If you can convince "splitters" (doctors who admit patients to other hospitals) to admit more of their patients in your facility, you can greatly expand the patient base with very little additional effort. Sometimes, all that is needed is a word of encouragement or appreciation. It may be necessary, however, to buy new equipment, improve facilities, make changes in nursing, or fix production problems before you get more admissions from a splitter. It is usually easier to get more business from existing customers than to find new customers. You should carefully monitor the admitting behavior of each physician, note any changes, and act to improve the situation. Even if you are not hospital-based, you need to be actively involved in bringing more business into your organization. In a sense, you should view yourself as a professional sales person. You are selling your organization and its products to potential buyers. You may no longer be involved in manufacturing (the direct provision of patient care), but you should be involved in strategic planning, quality assurance, cost reduction, productivity improvement, marketing, sales, and advertising.

The physician executive knows he or she is doing the job if the quality of care in the organization is improving. You are a major control point for quality assurance, and, if quality deteriorates, it is your fault. You should also be involved in determining quality standards and in setting specifications for computer systems that monitor quality of care. Have you made a major contribution to the risk management program?

Problem solving and decision making are traditional management functions. What organizational problems have you solved in the past 12 months? Have you studied and improved the way your organization makes decisions? If you can streamline medical care decision making in your organization, you are accomplishing an important job function. This may require intensive work with the medical staff, redesign of staff committees, or the development of a new corporate structure for physicians.

Better management of patient care is also an outcome that should be traceable to you. Providing patient care is a production process, and you should view yourself as a production manager.

It is important that you periodically assess physician, nursing, and patient satisfaction with the production process. Are waiting times too long? Is there confusion regarding referrals? Are procedures inefficient? Is documentation of patient care inadequate? Are the nursing units understaffed or overstaffed? Are admitting and discharge procedures quick and painless? You should diagram the flow of production in each patient care unit, with the times, procedures, and costs carefully noted. You may have to buy a stopwatch and do a little management engineering to determine if you have optimal production efficiencies. In our current reimbursement environment, a dollar saved is a dollar earned. Productivity improvement can offset eroding profit margins.

Another index of your performance is the quality of relationships you maintain with third parties. Do outside companies like to do business with your organization? In addition to being a physician, you must fulfill the roles of diplomat, negotiator, and public relations representative for your organization. It is important to maintain the right image and to facilitate working relationships with outside parties.

Physician satisfaction with your role in the organization and an absence of problems in your assigned areas of medical responsibility are important indicators that you are doing your job well. You are hired to solve problems, not create them. A well-organized and well-functioning group of physicians is a tribute to your capacity as a physician executive.

Are you successful in your attempts to recruit and retain physicians? If this is part of your job description, it is an outcome that should be measured. The right age and mix of the medical staff is important to the survival of your organization.

Innovation is an important organizational outcome and should be part of your performance appraisal. Have you developed new medical services and products for your organization? Have you increased the organization's service area? Have you developed profitable joint ventures? Have you designed an innovative new organizational structure for physicians working with your organization?

Is the community experiencing an improved community health status as the result of your work? This is a difficult performance objective to measure, but it is the reason your organization exists. Your attention to wellness and prevention services is an important step in reducing morbidity indices in your community.

Career Development

A physician executive must learn to manage his or her career. Your destiny depends on how well you function and progress in organizations. You need to develop a career strategy and plan that is reviewed and updated each year. You must know three things to be a good career planner:

- Where you are presently in your career.
- Your career destination.
- A plan for getting from here to there.

It may pay you to get some help from a career planner or to attend a career workshop. There is a large body of literature in this field, and you will benefit from some directed reading.

Don't stay in a bad organizational space. If the organization or the job does not fit you, get out! You will lose time and confidence fighting a losing battle. Remember, a good manager in a bad organizational space is a failure. Even if you can get by, you are losing opportunities to make valuable contributions to the field. Many physicians have never had occasion to resign or have never been fired. They feel that if they are having trouble, it must mean that something is wrong with them. That is a possibility. Another answer is that the fit between the job space and the physician executive is wrong. The only way to know for sure is for the physician executive to leave and seek greener pastures elsewhere.

Develop a professional network. Each time you attend a professional meeting, make contacts and collect business cards. You should have dozen or more peers with whom you regularly consult and share information. The best jobs come through professional networks. Often one of your peers has solved problems that stump you and, if asked, will be happy to share the solution with you.

Maintain a high visibility in your profession. You should be a member of the American College of Physician Executives. You should complete the Physician in Management Seminar offered by ACPE. You should attend the national meetings of ACPE. This builds a valuable network of contacts. If people do not know you, they can hardly help you.

Accept offices in national health organizations and serve on their committees. The practice is time-consuming, but it develops contacts and gives you valuable information not available to others in your profession. Remember, as a manager, you manage a knowledge base and you manage through the efforts of others. You have to stay in the mainstream to best serve your own interests and the interests of your organization.

Continue your formal and informal education. It may pay you to go for an MBA or an equivalent degree in management. The MD/MBA combination is a powerful vocational ticket. How much more education makes sense for you will depend on how many more years you plan to work as a physician executive.

Redesign your job. You can enrich your job and increase your satisfaction by adding new job elements that represent your special interests and abilities. Think about your ideal job space. If you could have it all, what would it be? Know what you need from your organization to be at your best.

Carefully analyze your successes and failures. Every manager learns from intelligent mistakes. Debrief your actions. Why did I win? Why did I lose? What will I do differently next time?

Good managers have a lot of experience and have made a lot of mistakes getting it. Unless you are willing to take risks and make mistakes, you will not learn. It is important that you work for an organization that will back you and take risks with you. No manager wants to be out on a limb.

Present papers at national meetings and contribute to the literature on physicians in management. As I indicated earlier, most management literature is not directed to your profession and is not easily adapted. If your writing skills are not up to par, work with a freelance writer. You will be the author, and the freelancer will prepare your manuscript for publication. A test of any professional is the degree to which he or she contributes to the literature of his or her profession.

Do not be afraid to file your credentials with one of the many professional search firms. You are worth to your organization what you are worth to other organizations. Determine your current market value and talk with the search firm concerning what you can do to make yourself even more attractive to other employers. Maintain an up-to-date personal resume and be certain that it has some recent additions to it.

You may want to develop your consulting skills both inside and outside your organization. Consultation is an important organizational development skill as well as a profession in its own right. What is there after being a physician executive—perhaps a consultant in physician management?

In general, it is good to be active in your community and to develop power bases outside your organization. You may wish to serve on the board of other community agencies and become active in community development. The more power and influence you have outside your organization, the more you have inside it.

Summary

As a physician executive, you are a key player on the management team. You are an interface professional spanning the disciplines of medicine and management. Your effectiveness in the organization depends on the appropriateness of your role definition and your possession of key management skills. This chapter has defined both of these. To further prepare yourself for success in your profession, consult the attached bibliography of current management literature. The bibliography is organized by topical area. Read in those areas where you will benefit most from further instruction. Although the selections are not written specifically for physician executives, you can easily adapt the material to your needs and interests. I have made no attempt to be exhaustive or necessarily representative of the vast literature available. I have instead included a few items in each topical area that I think will be of maximum benefit to you.

Leland R. Kaiser, PhD, is President of Kaiser and Associates, Brighton, Colorado. Dr. Kaiser holds an appointment as associate professor in the graduate program in health administration at the University of Colorado at Denver.

Chapter 3

Managing Physicians in Organizations

by Howard L. Kirz, MD, MBA, FACPE

The long-forgotten wag who first lamented that managing physicians was like "herding cats" would certainly have viewed the matter of this chapter with some skepticism, an oxymoron at best. In many ways, however, working with colleagues is at the very core of the work of physician executives in organizational settings. This chapter describes some of the major issues, some of the challenges, and some of the strategies for both successfully and happily fulfilling that work.

An Essential Value Conflict: Physicians in Organizations...Period!

One of the keys to working with physicians in any organizational setting is an empathy for and an understanding of the kinds of value conflicts a number of physicians face in all organizations these days. Articulating these conflicts, translating them into the context of professional values, and helping colleagues grapple with them are several hallmarks of the successful physician executive.

The first such conflict might simply be termed the "physician in organization" conflict or the Hobbesian conflict, named for Thomas Hobbs, who described the limits on individual freedom that occur as an inevitable part of membership in any society. Simply put, this conflict means that, to enjoy the benefits of membership in any given society, an individual gives up certain degrees of individual freedom and acquires in turn certain reciprocal rights and responsibilities. It may be one's individual right to drive drunk and blindfolded at 150 miles an hour somewhere on this globe, but not necessarily as a citizen of Washington and on the streets of Seattle.

The reciprocal to this limitation on individual freedoms in a society or an organization is the new right, and even a new responsibility, to be involved in developing the society's directions and norms. In other words to vote, to run for office, to lobby, to speak up, to participate as an enfranchised member of the society. The combination of these two phenomena, sometimes called the "social contract," describes the interdependent relationship between any individual and any society or, in our case, between any individual physician and a health care organization.

For some physicians in organizations, this conflict is felt as undeserved organizational encroachment on the individual "autonomy" thought to be an inherent professional right. Starr and others described this conflict in the '80s as part of the gradual transformation of American medicine from a cottage industry largely comprising independent individuals to a vastly more complex and interdependent one peopled and powered by organizations.[1] Since the 90's, particularly as health care reform creates even more complex organizations, this tension between individual professional rights and collective organizational rights has become part of the daily fare of most physicians and hence of most physician executives.

The limitations one experiences as a member of a defined medical organization and the reciprocal rights and responsibilities to help an organization define its norms and practice patterns are not necessarily obvious to individual physicians joining modern health care organizations. In fact, in some cases they're not even obvious to long-standing members of such organizations. And yet the two concepts, both the collective limitations and the needed contributions, are absolutely essential ingredients of the modern health care organization.

One of the first jobs of any physician manager in such a setting is therefore to help translate these general concepts into the specific professional milieu. To experience the numerous benefits of organizational life, not the least of which are a more certain flow of patients, an access to organizational services, and the use of the organizational franchise, individual physicians must accept both these limits and these responsibilities. It may for example be lawful and well within a physician's individual professional right to treat diabetics with coffee enemas somewhere on this globe, but not necessarily "on our enrollees," "in our hospital," or "as a member of our group practice."

As part of his or her daily work, the physician manager must be able to answer certain key questions that relate to these professional rights and limitations. What exactly are the benefits of professional membership or employment in this organization? What exactly are the limitations on professional autonomy to be expected as a member of this organization?

Why? How can an individual physician participate in the development of group norms, practice expectations, practice guidelines, benefit packages, organizational strategies? What are the responsibilities of the individual physician for participating in such activities? Why? What are the expectations of individual physicians for doing other kinds of organizational work? Why? How are professional disputes resolved here? What are the rights of the individual physician in this process?

Although this "individual in the organization" conflict has its origin in the roots of civilized society, many physicians will first experience the conflict as a provider within one or another modern health care organizations. Helping colleagues understand these essential tradeoffs, dealing with the resultant tensions, and empathizing with the dilemma are thus key characteristics of the successful physician manager in any organizational setting.

More Values in Conflict: Kantian Versus Utilitarian Ethics

As if the foregoing weren't enough, a second major conflict for physicians in many health care organizations today involves the physician's obligations to an individual patient versus obligations to a served population. "Traditional" (at least post-World War II and post-third-party insurance) Twentieth Century medical ethics holds that the physician must do everything possible for the potential benefit of each individual patient, so-called Kantian ethics. Such ethics are relatively without conflict in a world of seemingly unlimited resources and uncontested medical truths. In such a world, the question of individual versus population outcomes can be viewed largely as a philosophical exercise or at least as one restricted to physicians practicing in "managed care" organizations.

In the '90s, however, the era of apparently unlimited resources came to a grinding halt, and many more organizations have since adopted the dual mission of providing high-quality health care within defined fiscal limits. Operating within such defined resources requires the organization and its physicians to continually seek the most cost-effective and care-effective strategies for achieving a given health outcome. It likewise requires difficult resource allocating decisions that often balance the health needs of one group of patients against the needs of the population as a whole.

Such organizational missions put practicing physicians in the unaccustomed position of simultaneously caring for individual patients while being guardians of the best use of organizational resources for the care of an entire population. Organizational policies, such as expectations for length of stay, indications for certain procedures, allocation of scarce capital, and the deployment of support personnel, all place the physician potentially at odds with traditional medical ethics. As national and local health reform initiatives create more organizations with these missions, a growing number of American physicians will find themselves grappling with such conflicts.

Besides these kinds of resource allocation conflicts, a number of previous medical "truths" have come under scrutiny through the emerging sciences of outcomes analysis and population-based research. How good is the evidence that the health of an individual mother or child is actually improved by the old truth that one C-section should always beget another? Does doing more hysterectomies really have a positive impact on the health of the population? If not, what are the indications and ethical requirements for recommending one to an individual patient? What about skull films in trauma? Do they add anything but cost to patient outcomes in minor head injuries? Does routine PSA screening improve the health status of men aged 50-75, or does it actually decrease it?

There are, of course, no easy answers to these ethical and scientific dilemmas, but it often falls to a physician manager to help colleagues deal with these conflicts in an organizational setting. This work typically includes regularly articulating the source of such conflicts in our limited resource world; actively involving physicians in organization-level decision making about such matters; translating abstract organizational policies into practical medical ones understandable at the level of departments and practices; helping colleagues find rational solutions for the care of their individual patients; and accepting personal responsibility for resolving these individual care dilemmas when absolutely necessary.

As managing the health of populations within available resources becomes increasingly the charge of American health care, the work of individual physician executives will increasingly include this kind of ethical and scientific conflict resolution. Such work, although difficult, carries with it the considerable reward of helping colleagues thrive professionally and emotionally in our dramatically changing health care environment.

Teaching the Organization's Mission and Values

While translating and helping resolve the two conflicts described above is now part of the daily fare of virtually all physician leaders, it is the regular teaching and inculcation of an organization's basic mission and core values that offers the most successful preventive approach to managing physicians in organizational settings. Such teaching is equally relevant whether at the level of the organization itself or at the level of an individual department or facility within it.

The mission of any health care organization or any subunit should answer three key questions: "Whom do we serve" (who are our customers)? "Why" (for what purposes)? "How" (with what range of products or services)? Clarity about these questions allows physicians, nurses, managers, and other members of the health care team to come together around a sense of common purpose. It provides an answer to the basic workplace question: "What are we all doing here?" From the point of view of a physician executive, it also begins to lay the groundwork for a set of common professional expectations within the organizational context.

Defined values add greater detail to a mission by describing the most important beliefs of people working in the organization. Common examples might include the values of teamwork, cost effectiveness, defined levels of profit or growth, service quality to patients or enrollees, coordination between primary and secondary care, and active contribution to the community. Each of these explicitly stated values helps create a more consistent organizational culture and a clearer sense of appropriate behavior within the organization.

The physician executive has two important roles regarding mission and values. One is to teach, explain, and inculcate the overall organizational mission and its values to physicians who join it. Such teaching not only helps create a sense of shared purpose and of professional expectations in the organization, but also can go a long way toward helping avoid future conflicts.

A second role for physician managers at the department or facility level is to help local groups create a unique sense of mission and values within the overall organizational context. While the organizational level mission and values form a useful backdrop to this work, most clinicians are best able to identify with these abstract notions when they relate directly to their own practice settings. In this way, the abstract concept of customers can become "referring primary care and emergency physicians in our three county area," and the concept of product line becomes "operative orthopedics for the hand and back."

Teaching of an organization's overall mission and values and facilitation of a similar sense at the level of departments or facilities represent two important tasks for physician managers in organizational settings. Such group work is the essence of binding individual practicing physicians to a common organizational purpose and provides a critical baseline for managing physicians in any organizational setting.

The "Six Dimensions of Performance"
(What Kinds of Physicians Do We Really Want?)

Not every physician should be in every type of health care organization. In fact, most physicians don't want to be in every type of health care organization. And certainly most organizations don't want every physician. The needs of a staff-model HMO, a network of community physicians, a hospital-based specialty practice, an academic medical center, a multispecialty group practice, and a military treatment facility can differ dramatically. Carefully defining the physician characteristics that best fit a given organization's needs is an important step to the subsequent management of physicians within the setting.

In general, health care organizations seek practitioners with specific characteristics in six clusters of behavior—the "six dimensions of performance." Although organizations vary in their specific needs, some general observations can be made about each of the six dimensions, regardless of organizational setting.

- High technical and professional quality of care.
- High quality of patient service.
- High productivity.
- Commitment to appropriate use of health care resources.
- Effective peer and co-worker relationships.
- Contributions to the organization and community.

Technical Quality of Care

Knowledge of one's medical discipline and the technical ability to perform its clinical procedures are, of course, fundamental to the provision of excellent medical care. All physicians in an organization must possess technical and cognitive skills necessary for professional competence in their chosen specialty. In recent graduates, this is commonly demonstrated by the completion of the requisite residency, fellowship, or board certification. In the case of practicing physicians, a more detailed definition of appropriate procedural and cognitive skills required may be necessary. Credentialing and recredentialing processes are commonly used that detail these expected skills and competencies. As quality of care data systems become more sophisticated, organizations can increasingly define the desired technical quality in terms of procedure rates, complication rates, and direct patient outcomes. Every practitioner in an organization should be engaged in continuous self-education to maintain and upgrade these skills.

Quality of Service

The personal interaction between physician and patient to a great degree determines the level of satisfaction patients have with their health care and often with the organization itself. It is vital that patients find the "bedside manner" of their practitioners and support staff respectful, caring, and oriented to their needs. Although every member of the health care team affects a patient's perception of quality, it is the physician who can be most influential in both setting team norms and determining ultimate patient perception. Physicians should be expected to listen well and to clearly communicate their findings and plans to their patients. A number of organizations have developed detailed descriptions of the type of service behaviors they expect from their professional staffs. These expectations can include appointment and office wait times, patients' satisfaction with information received, explanations given, and even the physician's listening and respecting behaviors. A variety of organizational studies have demonstrated that patients and enrollees value quality of service at least as much as the technical quality of their care.

Practice Management Skills and Productivity

Modern health care organizations depend more and more on their ability to use every resource wisely. One measure of resource use is the output gained per unit of labor input—good old-fashioned productivity. In the purely fee-for-service world of the past, desired physician productivity could be fairly easily defined in terms of billings. With the onset of salaried physicians, capitation, and a variety of new organizational forms, definitions of expected physician productivity have become much more complex. Most definitions today, depending on the capabilities of the organization's encounter-tracking system, continue to include some measure of direct services provided—e.g., total billings, visits, procedures, relative value units, etc. Expected hours of work or total hours of patient availability (including call hours) are another common component. Panel sizes have become important in defining productivity expectations for primary care physicians.

Alongside such number counts, certain productivity-enhancing behaviors can also be defined. These include efficient scheduling practices, effective management of office staff, effective use of physician extenders, taking thorough responsibility for a defined population, and ensuring adequate backup or coverage for patients when unavailable.

Resource Utilization

Organizations today must be concerned about the most effective and appropriate use of all their health care dollars. Although physician labor costs represent only about 21 percent of total health care costs in the United States, physician behavior has a significant impact on other costs through styles of practice and through decisions about the use of other health care resources. With improved utilization- and quality-tracking systems, many organizations are attempting to describe desired physician utilization behavior with quantitative measures, such as average lengths of stay, costs per episode of care, referral rates, procedure rates, pharmacy costs, and overall utilization "profiles."

Because medical science is still so uncertain and because the sources of variation in most utilization data are vague, some organizations also define expected physician behaviors that will contribute to the most effective use of resources in any data milieu. These characteristics include a comfort with both the use and the limitations of such data, an interest in self-evaluation, a willingness to work with colleagues in the examination of utilization and quality data, and a commitment to the continuing search for best overall clinical strategies.

Peer and Co-Worker Relationships

An organization is, by definition, a complex interdependency of individuals working together to achieve a common purpose. Teamwork is critical to providing the very best and most efficient care. In all organizational settings, physicians must therefore be willing and able to work with a variety of others. These include departmental colleagues, referring and referral physicians, hospital and office nurses and support staff, and managers at a variety of levels. Physicians have a great impact on the workplace environment. Communication with peers and co-workers needs to be clear and respectful, and the ability to participate on and lead teams is frequently important.

Organizational/Community Contributions

Organizations are not composed of paper, steel, and brick alone. They require the continuous involvement of both groups and individuals in order to grow, thrive, and improve. For organizational physicians, this kind of involvement means more than just caring for one's patients and going home. It includes expectations for such activities as participation at medical staff and committee meetings, presentations at educational sessions and case reviews, involvement on quality improvement teams, working on clinical guidelines or organizational policies, and sometimes taking chairships or leadership positions. While the specific activity of individual physicians may vary with their interests and skills, a common expectation is that physicians will spend on the order of 10 percent of their time contributing in some way to the organization's growth and improvement.

In a like fashion, an organization exists within a geographic and professional community. Relationship to that community is important to the organization's success. Hence, physicians and other professional staff are frequently expected to participate in the community's activities. Local medical and specialty societies, charitable and political organizations, academic medical centers, schools, and sports teams are common examples. Some organizations desire professional publication, outside teaching, or research contributions from their professional staffs as well.

These six dimensions of performance form a basis for describing desired physician characteristics and for setting specific physician performance expectations in organizational settings. While organizations may vary in the exact characteristics they seek within each dimension, the overall template can be used in virtually any health care organization.

Carefully refining these specific professional expectations at a given organization usually involves the physician executive's doing group work with colleagues. This work can be done at both organizational and departmental levels. Few activities are as high yield. Simply getting colleagues together to begin to discuss common expectations has a strong effect on building the sense of group culture and organizational commitment. Detailed discussion of performance expectations helps clarify the sense of group direction and commonly reveals both existing and missing sources of data and support. Additional discussion generates understandable measures of performance. And finally, the definitions achieved through such work will prove invaluable in the subsequent steps of recruiting the right physicians to the organization; periodically reviewing physician performance, performance feedback, and coaching; and, when needed, managing marginal performance.

Recruiting and Selecting the Right Physicians at the Beginning

The initial "fit" between physician characteristics and organizational characteristics is one of the most important single determinants of subsequent physician satisfaction and performance. Developing and maintaining a recruiting process that ensures this fit is well worth the time.

Organizational recruiting begins with some prework, the most important aspect of which is a clear description of the kind of physician being sought. The "six dimensions" provide a useful template for such a description. Done in advance, this work can have a significant effect on the whole recruiting process.

Besides the six dimensions describing organizational expectations, the prework for recruiting should address issues related to the specific practice itself. This is sometimes called a "clinical job description." Common features in the clinical job description include the patient population served; common or special health conditions cared for; specific experience, skills, or certification needed; expectations regarding time commitment, work location, and schedule; hospital affiliation or privileges required; equipment, space, and personnel support available; contract, salary, benefits, and other financial arrangements; and the expected timeline for hiring. The next step in recruiting is what professional recruiters call "sourcing," i.e., generating an adequate pool of candidates. For most organizations, this is best viewed as an ongoing process rather than one triggered by an acute hiring need.

Examples of ongoing activities might include regular relationships with regional residency programs, local and national peer networking by professional staff, and periodic publications in professional journals. More acute sourcing strategies include advertising in selected professional journals, direct contacts with referred physicians, and the use of professional recruiters. "Cold calling," while common among securities salesmen and rug cleaners, has little place in professional recruiting.

Application forms should collect the basic information about experience, training, references, and other professional activities. The application process also provides some unique opportunities to explore questions about the possible fit between the candidate and the organization. Questions can be asked about virtually any of the six dimensions, about why this particular organization is of interest, and about previous experience in similar settings. Application materials and reference-checking can then be used to establish a first cut of candidates likely to thrive in the specific organizational setting.

With position requirements and organizational expectations in hand, a prescreening based on the application materials and reference checking can be accomplished, and an interview process can then be planned. The purpose of the interview is to accomplish three things: to elicit additional information from the candidate to help determine the fit, to provide the candidate with more information to help with his or her decision, and to begin the bridge to a potential long-term relationship. Good recruiting interviews are mutual exchanges in which both parties seek and learn information about the other. In conducting an interview, physician executives should explore how closely the values, philosophy, and goals of the individual match those of the organization. Good interviews likewise give candidates every opportunity to understand what joining this particular organization will mean to them. Ample time during the interview process should be made available to serve both needs.

When applications have been reviewed and interviews are completed, the selection process begins. Key questions are asked by the physician executive or selection committee. Are there ideal candidates who perfectly fit the organization's needs and expectations? Is the organization prepared to meet their needs and expectations? For candidates who, if not ideal, seem good fits overall, are the areas of risk or uncertainty acceptable? What should be done to minimize any of these uncertainties?

The physician executive can make a significant contribution to an organization's well-being by developing and managing a successful physician recruiting and selection process. Few decisions are as long-lasting as those about members of an organization's professional staff. A poor fit during this process rarely becomes a good one years later.

Orienting New Physicians

When expectations are clear and physicians are hired to fit those expectations, the orientation of new physicians to an organizational setting is a natural bridging process. If the first two steps are not completed well, physician orientation can easily become a conflict-ridden and frustrating activity.

The orientation of new physicians should follow closely on the heels of recruiting. Although the physician executive may not be personally appropriate to orient every new physician, he or she should ensure that the values and expectations discussed during recruiting are rediscussed during orientation, with additional specifics that address the particular practice setting.

In addition to the usual familiarization with people, forms, and places, physician orientation should include detailed information on clinical practice expectations. What quality measures are in use in this practice? How are clinical guidelines established here? What forums exist for involvement in developing these guidelines? How does the organization define and measure patient satisfaction? What are the exact productivity and practice management expectations here? What about expectations for work scheduling, case management, patient wait times, and utilization? What are the specific opportunities and expectations for the physician to contribute to the department, to the organization, and to the community?

A number of organizations use mentoring with a senior physician as a way to help new physicians acclimatize to organizational life. This technique is particularly useful during the first months in helping new physicians to interpret and deal with organizational norms for clinical practice. Many a recently hired physicians has found one timely bit of "how-I-really-do-it" advice worth reams of reading and days of touring.

Information for Periodic Performance Review

Health care organizations today often track large amounts of financial and utilization data for use in evaluating aspects of organizational performance. In addition, a number of organizations are developing improved means for measuring and tracking health care quality, including complication rates, clinical outcomes, and patient and enrollee satisfaction. Such systemic data can be invaluable for managing aspects of an organization's performance. To be truly useful in the management of individual physicians, it must be both accurate and interpretable to the physicians themselves. The role of a physician executive in this regard is to ensure that the organization's data systems meet these tests.

The conversion of aggregate data into usable information for individual performance management involves several steps. Accuracy of the separate data elements is an absolute requirement. No information system that relies on imprecise coding, incomplete capture of financial data, or inappropriate measures of quality can be reliably used for physician performance purposes. A second requirement is involvement of the organization's physicians directly in the design and formatting of data that will eventually be used in measuring their performance. This step, taken early in the evolution of such systems, not only will help develop data formats that feel and actually are understandable to clinicians, but also can go a long way toward dispelling some of the mistrust that inevitably surrounds such systems. Physician managers who take the time to involve clinical colleagues at this early point can avoid much later confusion and conflict trying to interpret data that make little sense at the level of actual practice.

Finally, to be truly useful, this kind of aggregate data needs both a denominator and a comparator appropriate to the organizational setting. In other words, visits per week may be an interesting productivity widget, but visits per defined age-sex-health status-adjusted panel makes it interpretable in a managed care setting. Likewise, the presence of a predetermined comparator (or "benchmark") is what allows one to interpret performance in the light of some predefined organizational expectation.

Besides these systemic data systems, a variety of less quantitative information sources typically exist that can be useful in measuring other dimensions of physician performance. Examples include patient complaints and compliments, co-worker and colleague perceptions, quality assurance reports, PRO and malpractice cases, and the self-reporting of community and educational activities. Behavioral surveys are likewise in frequent use as a way to periodically gather information about peer and co-worker relationships and about service quality. The key with this kind of information, as with systemic data, is the accuracy, relevance, and interpretability of the data at the level of the individual practitioner.

Feedback and Coaching

Giving and receiving effective feedback is an essential part of the physician executive's skill set for managing professional colleagues. Research shows that, to be effective, feedback must be individual-specific, understandable, accurate, and made available in a timely, facilitative, nonjudgmental manner. Feedback in health care organizations can take one of three forms: systemic, intermittent personal, and periodic personal.

Systemic feedback consists simply of making available to individual practitioners financial and quantitative data produced by the organization's aggregate data systems on a regular basis. Common systemic feedback includes production reports, utilization rates, and regular measures of technical and service quality. As described above, the primary role of physician executives providing this kind of feedback is to ensure that the data are accurate, relevant, and interpretable at the level of the individual provider and that clinicians have been appropriately involved in their design and formatting.

Intermittent personal feedback consists of staying alert to episodic data, activities, and behavior within a department or an organization and seeking opportunities to provide timely and personal feedback based on it. The atmosphere of receptivity toward such feedback is significantly enhanced by the physician executive's own openness to receiving it. Intermittent personal feedback is most effective when it is behaviorally specific and when it relates observed behavior to that expected in the organization. In this way, feedback about an episode of loud public verbal abuse of a receptionist becomes less a debate about scheduling glitches and more a discussion of respectful relationships with co-workers.

Intermittent personal feedback can be especially useful when it focuses on the positive. When the physician executive catches a colleague "doing something right" and tells him or her about it, the effects can be extraordinary. Physicians, like other organizational staff, often feel a lack of appreciation for their contributions. Physicians respond quite well to a colleague's recognition of their work and also to understandable and behavior specific observations that can help them do their jobs better. In the busy life of a physician executive, it may be difficult to remember this aspect of the job, but a few personal experiences have convinced many experienced physician leaders to spend the time needed to provide this important personal feedback to colleagues and co-workers.

Periodic personal feedback is typically part of a formal periodic performance review and is often part of the organization's annual review process for its professional staff. Such periodic reviews provide a regularly scheduled opportunity for face-to-face dialog between the physician executive and individual physicians.

Done perfunctorily or with a judgmental attitude, periodic performance review can easily become a source of dissatisfaction to the individual physician and a significant waste of time for the physician executive. On the other hand, physician managers who are open to reciprocal feedback and who use a facilitative and constructive approach can achieve excellent results.

The manner in which data are presented and discussed during periodic performance review significantly affects their reception. Facilitative, constructive feedback is descriptive. It provides a verbal picture, not a judgment. Instead of adjectives, opinions, and conclusions ("I guess you're just getting a little slower with age"), data are presented in clear, specific, and limited fashion ("On this report, your total visits are 15 percent lower than last year's"). Such an approach lends itself to mutual exploration and learning. Judgmental approaches impede the feedback process and inhibit learning by both parties.

Physician executives who use periodic personal feedback most effectively neither blame or judge; they simply provide the data clearly and make themselves available to help with the data's interpretation. The cause of apparent performance variations is often not known to either party to the feedback until it is examined together. Mutual exploration of the available data without one-way analysis helps produce a neutral, open environment in which both parties can learn. Excessive interpretation by the physician manager, highly judgmental conclusions in any direction, and overreading the significance of minimal data are three common causes of failure of periodic feedback.

The notion of "coaching" captures the appropriate style for providing feedback to professional colleagues very well. Drucker has said that the essence of the coaching attitude is the simple question, "What can I do to help you be the best you can be?"[2] A coaching attitude acknowledges both the professional competence of the physician and the physician manager's appropriate role in jointly examining the data and in supporting any desired changes.

Performance Improvement and Managing Marginal Performance

Appropriate recruiting, clear definitions of expected behavior, accurate and interpretable information, effective feedback, and a coaching style are important tools in the armamentarium of managing physicians. Given most physicians' inherent intelligence and desire to do well, these tools are the most frequently used in helping colleagues succeed in the organizational environment.

Occasionally, however, these approaches fail, and physician behavior continues at a level and type that falls significantly below the organization's expectations. When such a problem occurs over time and is not corrected despite routine feedback and coaching, it may be termed "marginal performance." It is clearly one of the most difficult and emotion-laden management problems facing any physician executive.

Marginal performance, although rare, may occur in any of the six dimensions of physician performance. Although the frequency of each type of problem varies with organizational setting, the most common examples of marginal performance would include problems with peer and co-worker communications, patient satisfaction, technical quality of care, utilization of services, and productivity. In all health care settings, the behavioral consequences of substance abuse, depression, or physical illness can first appear as chronic performance problems.

A common approach to dealing with these significant performance discrepancies is the use of a "performance improvement planning" process. This approach begins with an explicit description of the desired behavior or outcome and a clear statement of the way in which actual behavior differs. It then moves to a mutual exploration of the possible causes of this discrepancy and a joint agreement on the actions to be taken by the two parties in resolving it.

Sometimes, obstacles are found that actually inhibit the physician's ability to perform as expected (e.g., inadequate office support). In these instances, the physician executive must frequently be willing to assist with the solution. Sometimes, educational or skill deficiencies surface that may require time or money to correct. Sometimes, the problem will be one of volition or lack of intent to change behavior.

Using a performance improvement approach, the next step is to negotiate a "contract" for change. What exact actions are expected? What supporting acts will be taken by the physician manager? How exactly will change be monitored? What will be the consequences of improvement? What exactly will be the consequences of failure to improve? When will the two parties next meet?

The components of a formal performance improvement process should always be captured in writing. This documentation must include a clear description of the expected behavior, data describing the discrepancy in actual behavior, dates and times of previous feedback, and all aspects of the "contract." The contract portion should include a description of the responsibilities of each party, the monitors, the dates of review, and the consequences of various results.

The need for a formal process is thankfully rare in dealing with professional colleagues. When needed, however, it can be essential to fair and measured management of significant performance discrepancies. In experienced hands, it can be expected that half or more of discrepancy problems will improve with such an approach. Continued monitoring and support for the change is often necessary.

When all else fails, the final option available to managing serious, unremitting performance deficiencies is use of the organization's process for involuntary adverse action. These processes, which vary by type of organization, are governance actions that unilaterally limit or terminate the relationship between the health care organization and the physician. Examples include contract termination, limitation or termination of privileges, termination of employment, limitation of work conditions, etc.

The use of such drastic measures depends in all but the most acute circumstances on the previously described foundation of data, feedback, coaching, and performance improvement. With an adequate foundation, adverse action can be effectively and fairly employed as a "fail-safe" in cases of unresolvable performance problems. Such actions are never pleasant or easy, but they must occasionally be taken in the best interests of patients, the organization, or the other professional staff.

Summary

Managing physicians is at the very heart of successful medical management in the organizational setting. Not only are physician behaviors essential to the provision of high-quality health care; they directly affect customer service perceptions, utilization rates and the cost of care, and the team and collaborative atmosphere essential for long-term success.

To develop an environment in which these things can occur with fellow physicians, the physician manager has many tools. Empathy for and assistance with the value conflicts experienced by many physicians in health care organizations is an important first ingredient. Facilitating, building, and teaching a sense of common purpose, mission, and values, at both organizational and subunit levels, is essential. Health care organizations and the physician executives within them need to clearly define what behaviors are expected of their professional staffs in at least six dimensions of performance. Armed with this clarity and clinical job descriptions, recruiting activities have a higher likelihood of finding physicians for whom the organizational environment will be a good professional and personal fit. Orientation procedures can further improve this sense of fit. Regular feedback of accurate and interpretable data and periodic review of performance with a positive, coaching style are strategies well suited to working with intelligent and highly motivated professional team members.

Occasionally, when behaviors or outcomes fall below well-defined organizational expectations, a behavioral contracting model can be used to assist with marginal performance. Rarely, the fail-safe of adverse disciplinary action must be taken to protect patients and the organization.

Managing physicians is a complex, sometimes frustrating, and always important aspect of the role of physician executives. Done well, however, few activities can make so much positive difference to the well-being of the health care organization, its patients, and its professional staff.

References

1. Starr, P. *The Social Transformation of American Medicine.* New York, N.Y.: Basic Books, 1982.

2. Drucker, P. *Management: Tasks, Responsibilities, Practices.* New York, N.Y.: Harper & Row, 1973.

Other Reading

Allenbaugh, G. "Coaching...A Management Tool for a More Effective Work Performance." *Management Review* 72(5):21-6, May 1983.

Brennan, E. *Performance Management Workbook.* New York, N.Y.: Prentice Hall, 1989.

Carter, L. and Lankford, S. *Physician's Compensation: Measurement and Benchmarking.* New York: Wiley and Sons, 2000.

Hargrave, J. *Strictly Business: Body Language.* Dubuque, Iowa: Kendall Hunt Publishing, August 2001.

Mager, R., and Pipe, P. *Analyzing Performance Problems.* Belmont, Calif.: Fearon Pitman Publishers, Inc., 1970.

McGregor, D. "An Uneasy Look at Performance Appraisal." *Harvard Business Review,* May-June 1957, pp. 133-138, Reprint #72507.

Porter, L. *Giving and Receiving Feedback; It Will Never Be Easy, But It Can Be Better.* NTL Reading Book For Human Relations Training. Alexandria, Va.: National Training Laboratory Institute, 1982.

Scholtes, P., and others. *The Team Handbook.* Madison, Wis.: Joiner Associates, 1988.

Howard L. Kirz, MD, MBA, FACPE, was Principal, the Clearwater Group, Bainbridge Island, Washington at the time this chapter was written. For many years prior to that time he served in various capacities with Group Health Cooprtative of Puget Sound, including its chief executive officer. Dr. Kirz died in 2008 of an unexpected heart attack.

Chapter 4

Developing a Competitive Marketing Strategy

by Eric Berkowitz, PhD

Over the past 30 years, the functional business discipline of marketing has become a basic component of a health organization's strategy. When first introduced in the 1970s, marketing was seen as a novel and in many ways negative aspect of a "business" influence for a health care organization. Marketing was viewed as advertising, and this sales-oriented approach was considered inappropriate in a professional environment involved with patients and their health status. In fact, many organizations today still struggle with the appropriate and full use of marketing within their strategies, and many health care professionals still resist utilization of marketing methods and concepts within their business plans. The purpose of this chapter is to discuss the meaning of marketing and how it affects the planning process of organizations, as well as the key components of marketing strategy formulation.

Marketing is both a process and a philosophy. In integrating marketing into an organization, the hospital or the medical group must view the service offering not from the perspective of the provider, but rather from that of the buyer. To be market-driven is to be customer-responsive. In its simplest form, marketing may be defined as the process by which customer needs are identified and a product (or service) is developed in response to those needs.[1] The service is delivered, priced, and promoted according to the best way to attract the consumer. Four components of strategy in this perspective of marketing—referred to as the four P's of marketing, or the marketing mix (product, price, place, and promotion)—will be discussed in greater depth in this chapter. All organizations have these four components in their control to some extent. That is, what products or services should be offered and at what price? How should these services be delivered or made accessible (place), and in what manner can the market be informed of the service's existence (promotion)?

The consumer is at the center of the marketing process. It is the consumer's needs to which the organization responds. For most health care organizations, this definition of the consumer varies and rarely consists of a single constituency. Figure 1, below, shows some of the multiple markets that exist for a hospital, a multi-specialty group practice, or a single program such as adolescent chemical dependency. The challenge for health care organizations in developing an effective marketing approach is balancing the often varying needs of each market with the respective clinical service quality issues of the provider.

Figure 1. Multiple Markets/Multiple Providers

Provider	Markets
Hospital	Patients Physicians Corporations HMOs
Multispecialty Group	Patients Physicians Corporations
Adolescent Chemical Dependency Program	Parents Judges Social Workers Third-Party Payers

The Market-Driven Planning Sequence

Recognizing that marketing is driven by the consumer has a significant implication for the planning process of the organization. Historically, health care organizations were not market-driven. Rather, planning occurred from an internal perspective. In the typical planning mode, the hospital or group might examine statistics on the market in terms of age or income, along with various epidemiological data of primary and secondary service areas. The confluence of these factors might lead to a decision that a particular service was or wasn't needed in the community. After commitment to the development of the service, it was left to the administrator or chief financial officer to determine pricing for the service. No formal strategy was developed for the service beyond offering this new program. Scheduling, location of the satellite facility, or determination of how the market would be informed of the service was left to the discretion of the providers of the service.

In a market-driven approach, introduction of a new service occurs as the result of a very different set of activities. Often, providers within a group or a hospital might suggest a new service, such as rehabilitation medicine or a scoliosis clinic. Before the service is rolled out, an assessment of the market is made. Is there a demand for this new service? Are there other providers in the market? What price are buyers willing to pay for this offering? Where would users like to receive this service and during what hours? In a market-driven sequence, the definition of a service is really provided by the likely buyer or user of the service. The provider's role is to ensure clinical quality and to deliver the offering.

In considering the conditions that existed for most health care organizations up to the mid-1970s, it is easy to understand why a market-based approach was never integrated into typical health care planning. For most of the 1950s, 1960s, and even 1970s, most communities were still underserved with regard to a range of clinical services or providers. In fact, for most hospitals and other medical institutions, this period was not one of great cost or utilization pressure. When a service was offered, the primary problem was typically that of trying to meet demand rather than to stimulate it. In the rare instance in which a medical organization offered a new service that was not successful, it was often viewed by the board of trustees or physicians as a good learning experience. Why is a marketing-based approach now a more common occurrence? Rarely is the problem now facing medical organizations one of meeting demand. It is more likely a situation of trying to generate utilization or volume. Additionally, 15 or 20 years ago, most health care organizations were in relatively strong financial positions. A new clinical service that was not successful financially *could* be seen as a learning experience. Today, there are few health care organizations that can afford very many learning experiences.

The importance of a market-driven approach is being recognized among medical groups that have ventured into extended hour programs or weekend appointment schedules. Often, these programs are tried because a particular physician in the group has gone to a conference and heard that other medical groups are offering weekend hours. After offering these hours, the group finds that the only thing accomplished was to increase the overhead of the organization and make the quality of life for the staff less desirable.

In using the market-based approach to planning, one would consider the offering of weekend hours or any new service by also determining whether it is for an offensive or defensive strategic purpose. For example, the organization should first survey consumers whom it would like to get as patients (but does not presently) and ask, "If the XYZ medical group were to offer weekend hours by appointment, how likely would you be to switch to it for your care?" That is, would the weekend hours increase business, an offensive strategy. Or, one might pose the question to existing patients whom the group wishes to maintain by asking, "If another medical group in the community were to offer weekend hours by appointment, how likely would you be to switch?" Is the group developing a market-driven strategy to retain a customer base, a defensive rationale?

The Keys to the Market Planning Approach

As one considers the market-driven planning approach, it is important to recognize three key aspects that significantly influence the resultant success of the planning sequence:

1. Utilization of marketing research in the early development stage of the plan and in pre-testing of the proposed program or service.

2. Development of a differential advantage

3. Definition of the target market

Using Marketing Research

In a market-driven planning approach, the role of marketing research occurs early in the process. At the beginning, it is marketing research that will help to identify service gaps patients might experience in their community regarding access to primary care, service referral deficiencies primary care providers might experience in terms of the tertiary centers that they presently use, or the ways in which companies might see more value from the health care plans they presently offer their employees. Later in the market-driven planning process, marketing research methodologies are particularly helpful in pre-testing the service proposal prior to its being offered. This aspect of marketing research will be discussed in greater detail after the varying marketing research methodologies are presented.

Marketing research data can be obtained in two broad ways—through the use of secondary data or primary data. Secondary data are data or information that was collected for some other purpose but is used in the analysis of the business problem at hand. For example, the U.S. Government collects census information that a company might well use for examining the demographic match of a community for the locations of a primary care clinic. Primary data are information that the health care organization collects for the particular question under consideration. For example, in developing a women's health program, the hospital conducts personal interviews with 300 women in the community.

Secondary Data

In health care, several secondary data sources too numerous to mention here are used.[2] However, some novel approaches have been developed by companies in the application of secondary data. One such company, Claritas (www.claritas.com/main.htm), combines census data with sociological and attitudinal profiling information by zip codes. This information has been used for target marketing, site location, and customer analysis. National research Corporation (www.nationalresearch.com) provides satisfaction measures; market analysis, and survey data for health care organizations.

With any secondary data sources, the health care organization must asked themselves some basic questions about the database:

1. How timely is the information?
2. How large and representative is the sample relative to the market that is relevant for the health care organization?
3. How free of bias are the data?
4. Are the data classified in a manner that is managerially useful for the organization?

Increasingly, with the advent of more sophisticated computerized programs and analysis techniques, organizations are turning to their own data and trying to create data warehouses. Data warehouses are an organization-wide centralized database of customer information. The organization can then utilize sophisticated data mining techniques to examine customer behaviors or patterns in order to further refine the health care organization's marketing strategy.[3]

Primary Data

Because of the limitations of secondary data, most organizations will collect primary data for a project of importance. Figure 2, page 56, shows common methods used in collecting primary data and the respective tradeoffs with each technique. Increasingly in health care, focus groups are seen as a valuable tool.[4]

In focus groups, a trained moderator leads 10-12 individuals through a series of relatively open-ended questions. While they do not provide empirical numbers, focus groups can often reveal issues and concerns that can be explored further in a mail or phone survey. Focus groups are increasingly used in two different steps in the marketing research process. Many organizations use them at the beginning of the research process to reveal issues, such as the possible reasons a radiology group isn't getting

Figure 2. Alternative Research Methodologies *

Research Methodology

Approach Criteria	Personal Interview	Telephone Survey	Mail Survey	Focus Groups
Economy	Most expensive.	Avoids interviewer travel, relatively expensive. Trained interviewers needed.	Potentially lower costs (if response rate sufficient).	Relatively expensive.
Interviewer bias	High likelihood of bias. Trust. Appearance.	Less than personal interviewer. No face-to-face contact. Suspicion of phone call.	Interviewer bias eliminated. Anonymity provided.	Need trained moderator.
Flexibility	Most flexible. Responses can be probed.	Cannot make observations. Assistance can be provided in completing forms.	Least flexible. Probing possible to a degree.	Very flexible.
Sampling and respondent cooperation	Most complete sample possible, with sufficient call back strategy.	Limited to people with telephones. No answers. Refusals are common.	Mailing list. Nonresponse a major problem.	Need close selection.

*Reprinted from Hillestad, S. and Berkowitz, E. Health Care Marketing Plans: From Strategy to Action. Second Edition. Rockville, Md.: Aspen Press, 1991, p. 100.

referrals. Or, focus groups can be used at the end of the research process to help explain the results in a survey. For example, a focus group might be constructed to better understand why 75 percent of responders indicated they were somewhat dissatisfied with the service of the emergency department. Focus groups are particularly useful in testing a program proposal prior to final implementation. In health care organizations, one cannot develop the service or the program without incurring significant costs in terms of physical space, the hiring of skilled clinicians, and related resource costs. As a result, in order to successfully pre-test it is important to develop a detailed concept description of the service—what it will include, what the charges will be, how patients or referral physicians might access the service, and other user dimensions. Examination of the detailed concept by a focus group can ensure that no aspect of the proposed program is missing a key component.

No doubt all readers have been at the receiving end of phone, mail, and personal interviews, so definitions of each approach aren't needed. However, a few comments about each methodology may be helpful. In conducting personal and telephone interviews, it is important to use trained interviewers. The potential for bias with an untrained interviewer can make data collection highly suspect. Phone interviews are also a very valuable way to collect information quickly.[5] Mail surveys are difficult to conduct because of non-response bias. While many methods are available for improving response rates for mail surveys, the ultimate question is always whether the person who responded is in any way different from the individual who did not respond. Except for the cost savings of mail surveys, there is little else to speak to their advantage beyond protection of the identity of the respondent.

In terms of the collection of primary data, the marketing research world is undergoing significant change. Organizations are increasingly turning to the creation of Web-based survey tools, such as those designed by Hosted Survey (www.hostedsurvey.com) and other companies.

Developing a Differential Advantage

A second key aspect of successful marketing is the development of a differential advantage. Often in health care, one hospital decides to open a pediatric emergency department, and the second hospital in the community opens its in response. Yet the second hospital does nothing that is in any way different from the first provider, and there is no resultant competitive advantage.

Organizations can turn to one of three places to establish a differential advantage—cost-based, product-based, or market-based.[6] In this framework, one might view Southwest Airlines and Kaiser Permanente as organizations that historically have positioned themselves as having a cost-based differential advantage. In a market-based differential advantage, one focuses on a narrow market segment (a geriatric medicine clinic) or on a defined geographic region. A product-based differential advantage has a real product or service difference. In the creation of any differential advantage, it is important to recognize the hallmarks of a "good" differential advantage. Foremost, it must be important to the buyer. An organization can do many things that are important and valuable, but the customer must value them. Second, a good differential advantage must be perceived by the buyer. A truism of marketing is that perception is reality. If the customer doesn't perceive the organization's clinical excellence, the organization does not have the excellence. The third component of a good differential advantage is that it must be unique. In a competitive market, this is almost the most difficult aspect of a differential advantage. It leads to the final criterion of a good differential advantage—it must be sustainable. In this last regard, the organization tries to create service or market advantages that are not easily copied by competing provider organizations.

Defining the Target Market and Market Segmentation

One other aspect of marketing and marketing strategy must be underscored in order for a market-based approach to planning to be effective— the target market. The term target market may be best defined as one or more specific groups of customers to whom an organization directs its strategy.[7]

Target Markets

Target markets were historically never a consideration in health care. When hospital CEOs were asked about their target markets, they often responded with data about the primary or the secondary service area or with a zip code analysis of admissions through the emergency department. When a physician establishes a practice, the office is opened and people who call or walk in are treated. In traditional marketing, the target market is an organizationally determined aspect of strategy. It is more a question of whom the organization wants to attract. It is important to recognize, in terms of marketing strategy, that the group of consumers that an organization attracts may be very different from whom it would like to get. It is the latter group that represents the target market. The market-based planning approach is aimed at members of this target market. Subsequent strategy is built around attracting the targeted population.

An important ethical comment must be raised around the entire issue of target markets in health care. The definition of a target market does not imply denying care to anyone who walks into the medical organization for treatment, but treating anyone who walks through the door is different from developing a strategy to go after a particular group of consumers. The four Ps discussed in the following pages are directed to a target market that is determined by the organization. Having determined the target market, the organization can begin to formulate a marketing strategy based on the four Ps.

Market Segmentation

A central concept drives marketing thinking—market segmentation. Market segmentation consists of identifying a subgroup of consumers in the population with similar wants and needs and tailoring the marketing mix to meet that subgroup's needs. The belief is that the closer the organization can tailor the marketing mix to an individual's preferences, the greater the likelihood that the individual will buy the product or service from that provider.

There are two traditional ways to segment the market. The first, sociodemographics, has been common in health care. Marketing is segmented by age, gender, income, or ethnicity. In health care, programs have been established in pediatrics, geriatrics, and women's health. Even income has been a form of segmentation in health care. The Washington Hospital Center has developed its Pavilion, a well-decorated area of the hospital with amenities such as heated towel racks, carpeting, specially prepared meals, and even a concierge service, to be targeted to the upscale patient.

A second way to segment has interesting implications for marketing strategy in a fee-for-service world and dramatic implications in a managed care world. This approach is referred to as heavy half segmentation. Heavy half segmentation is based on the principle that a small group of consumers tends to account for a disproportionate amount of a product's sales.[8] For example, 17 percent of all households account for 88 percent of all the beer sold; 39 percent of all households account for 90 percent of all soft drinks sold. A middle group of consumers account for the remaining percentage of product sales, and a large percentage of consumers do not buy the product at all.

The heavy half phenomenon has important marketing implications in health care. For example, in a fee-for-service world, a primary care practice will find that a large percentage of its patient revenue is generated from a relatively small number of charts. The important marketing goal in a fee-for-service environment is to retain these consumers. Prior to making any operational changes within the practice or a program, it is imperative to pretest the change with loyal consumers to ensure that they will not become alienated or dissatisfied. The key objective with consumers who use the practice but are not heavy users is to identify what can be done to make them loyal users. Is their use limited because they are healthy, or is it that they are splitting their care among providers? Finally, within any practice or health care organization's service area, a large number of consumers do not use the facility or practice at all. The major marketing question is to determine whether they do not use it because they have heard negative things about the facility or because they are loyal to other providers. Or, is their lack of use because of no knowledge of what the organization can offer them in terms of meeting their health care needs? This latter issue becomes a promotional challenge for marketing.

The heavy half segmentation perspective also has some interesting implications in a managed care world. Most managed care organizations would recognize that this segmentation scheme exists. A large percentage of the organization's utilization tends to come from a small percentage of subscribers. A middle group of subscribers accounts for most of the remaining utilization, which is not significant but is within the norms of health utilization statistics. Some subscribers join the plan but never use the practice during the contract period. From a marketing perspective, the objectives shift from a fee-for-service world. The heavy users are a group who must be served. To deny care to this group because they are a financial drain on the organization would be unethical and illegal. Yet, from a marketing perspective, the key challenge is to maintain the subscriber base of medium and nonusers. With the middle segment of subscribers, the goal is to ensure that they experience no service delivery failures when they interact with the organization. Because these occasional users have limited experience with the managed care plan, any service delivery failure may give them justification for switching to another plan when their contract renewal period occurs. The nonuser segment must be targeted in the last quarter prior to re-enrollment. These individuals should be contacted and should have some direct, personal interaction with the managed care entity. This interaction might consist of a health assessment or a brief health status discussion with a doctor. The reason is that, within 90 days, that person will be faced with a re-enrollment decision. That valued subscriber must have some sense of identity with the organization to ensure that he or she will not shift to a lower cost plan.

In recent years, there has been a third way to segment that is gaining popularity in marketing. It is based on cohorts—groups of individuals who were born during the same period of time and who have experienced significant events that shaped their values, attitudes, and approach to life. These events have been called "defining moments."[9] In the United States, seven distinct cohorts have been recognized: Depression Cohort, World War II, Post-War, Boomers I and II, and Generation X, and N Gen. Figure 3, page 61, shows the overall profile of the seven cohorts identified.

Figure 3. Cohort Profiles*

Cohorts	Years Born	Attitudes/Values
Depression	1912-1921	Practical, safety and security
World War II	1922-1927	Respect for authority
Post-war	1928-1945	Conservative, value stability
Boomer I	1946-1954	Individuality, question everything
Boomer II	1955-1965	Cynical
Gen X	1966-1976	Pragmatists, family
N Gen	1977-1984	Team players, respect for institutions

*Adapted from: Smith, J., and Clurman, A., Rocking the Ages, New York, N.Y.: Harper Business, 1997, and Meredith, G., Schewe, C., and Karlovich, J. Defining Markets, Defining Moments, New York, N.Y.: Hungry Minds Press, 2002.

While it requires more detail than can be presented here, the approach to looking at the market from a cohort perspective is gaining increasing popularity with marketers. The underlying premise of this segmentation scheme is that a person's values do not change as he or she ages. In health care, the implications are significant. The 65-year-old patient of today will not be the same as a 65-year-old patient 10 or 15 years from today. Members of the post-war cohort continue to be conservative or respect authority, and the boomers' values of individualism and questioning everything will not change as they age. Medical organizations will need to respond to the market not in terms of age as much as with regard to cohorts.

Product: The Foundation of Strategy

The focus of marketing strategy revolves around the product or service. In marketing, a central concept in developing the product or service strategy is the product life cycle. The product life cycle concept assumes that all products (or services) go through four distinct stages; introduction, growth, maturity, and decline. Figure 4, page 62, shows a generalized product life cycle curve. On the x-axis is time, and the y-axis represents sales or gross revenues. In each stage, market conditions change, which requires a change in organizational strategy. At the introduction stage, sales rise slowly. At growth, significant increases in sales occur. Sales level off during maturity. Ultimately, revenue drops during decline.

Figure 4. The Product Life Cycle

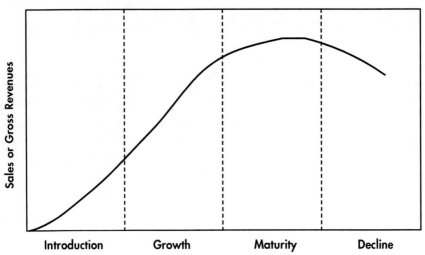

Introduction   Growth   Maturity   Decline

Introduction

In the introduction stage, the new service enters the market. For example, the first pediatric sports medicine program opens in the community. With regard to marketing strategy, there is one overriding objective in the introduction stage: to generate awareness of the new service. At this stage, promotion becomes important. Either advertising announcing the new service or strong personal sales efforts, such as informational lectures by physicians or others, are required to inform potential users of the service.

In terms of pricing decisions, there are two typical options at the introduction stage—skimming or penetration. In rolling out a new product or service, there are some distinct advantages to a low or penetration pricing strategy. Typically, this approach makes acceptance of the new service easier, because the buyer's financial risk is reduced. Also, it has the effect of delaying competitors from entering the market. Any new competitor must attempt to price lower, which is often difficult when facing a penetration pricing strategy. For many service businesses, however, this pricing approach is risky. When estimation of demand for a new service is somewhat difficult to accurately gauge, a penetration pricing strategy may lead to some organizational capacity problems. Demand can be greater than can be met through the staffing of the clinical service. While the organization is pleased at the market response, the delay in access to the new service can create ill will in the marketplace.

When capacity is an issue, it may be wise to price high (skimming). In this way, buyers who truly value the service will purchase it. The provider can gradually meet a larger potential demand by lowering prices as facility capacity expands. Skimming also allows the organization to recoup its often-high investment costs in setting up a new program before more aggressive price-cutting occurs as other competitors enter the market. In a service business such as health care, a high price also plays an important role in terms of image. For many buyers, a perceived price/quality relationship is often enhanced by a higher price. The major disadvantage of a high price is that it encourages competition to enter the market. Other providers, seeing the high price being charged for a particular service, may feel that they could enter the market, offer a program of similar quality, and be more attractive to the market by undercutting the higher priced alternative.

One other aspect of the introduction stage is essential from a marketing perspective. Product quality must meet customers' expectations. The quickest way to kill a new product is to offer it to the market before internal problems are worked out. For example, aggressive promoting of an industrial medicine program is essential in the introduction stage of the service's life cycle. However, if staffing problems or physical plant constraints or logistics have not been worked out, a market disaster is sure to occur. Corporations are attracted by the promotion of the new industrial medicine program. Salespeople sign contracts. Workers begin to show up for physicals, rehabilitation, or treatment for job-related injuries, and the health care organization does not have the resources or the capacity to meet the demand in a timely, efficient fashion. It is very unlikely that these dissatisfied buyers will be willing to sign contracts in the second year on the basis of assurances from the provider that the "kinks" have been worked out.

Being the first entrant into the market has the marketing advantage of being able to establish the market's expectation with regard to the product or service. The first entrant can set the price/value relationship of the particular program in the minds of the buyers.

Growth

The second stage of the product life cycle is the period of the most rapid increases in sales. It is in this stage that competitors enter the market. At the growth stage, the focus of attention becomes locking up the referral flow for patients. For new entrants at the growth stage, the key is to develop a differential advantage relative to the first provider. Typically, the source of the differential advantage is some aspect of the marketing mix. The second or third medical group to enter might offer extended hours or more satellite locations for its pediatric sports medicine program.

The issue of a differential advantage is a key concern once a competitor enters the market. The first entrant (the firm that began in the introduction stage) has the differential advantage of being first. The price that the first entrant pays in being first is primarily a promotional or an educational cost. That is, the first entrant must educate the market as to the value of a behavioral medicine program integrated within a primary care clinic or of a new approach to management or treatment of a particular disease. Each successive entrant must establish a differential advantage relative to the first. The four Ps are the place to turn, along with the target market selection, for a differential advantage. A later entrant could enter with a broader service line (the product component), more satellite facilities or extended hours (place), a lower premium per covered life (price), or better or more extensive advertising or public relations (promotion). Experience shows that it is often difficult to enter the market as a second or third entrant with a higher price. Additionally, promotion is a weak form of differential advantage, because the benefits are often temporal and transitory. Ideally, in terms of the four Ps, one might turn to the product or to distribution to establish a differential advantage of value to the market.

In addition to the four Ps, an organization can turn to the target market for a differential advantage. That is, the organization can tailor its program or services to a particular market segment, such as the high-income consumer or women. Women's health programs have been implemented by many facilities to establish a differential advantage with a comprehensive bundle of services for a particular market. As mentioned earlier, the Pavilion at the Washington Hospital Center is an attempt to establish a differential advantage with a specific set of upscale consumers.

Maturity

The third phase of the life cycle is when sales begin to level off. At this point, marginal competitors often will begin to leave the market. The focus of attention at this stage is to maintain market share. Because the market is mature, any lost customers will not be easily replaced. Customer retention is the key. At this point of the life cycle, it is important to look for new opportunities or service alternatives to get back up on the growth curve.

Decline

The final stage is the period of declining sales. At this stage, the organization typically must make the decision to drop the product or determine another efficient way of providing the service. In the past few years in certain markets, some hospitals have dropped obstetrics or pediatrics. Other hospitals, in an attempt to offer a service, have signed agreements to have the service provided by a third party. This stage is often the most difficult for companies to manage. In traditional industries, it is often believed that a disproportionate amount of management time and attention is spent in dealing with declining products.

Price: The Key to Revenue

As previously discussed, price plays an important role for an organization in setting the strategy for the introduction of a new service. It is important to recognize the difference between the marketing and the finance perspectives regarding price. In most health care settings, the issue of price is decided internally. That is, what are internal costs, the overhead allocation, and the margin? It is on the basis of these determinations, in conjunction with reimbursement constraints, that pricing decisions are made.

From a marketing perspective, these internal pricing concerns are important. But, in consideration of the external to internal perspective of marketing, it is the market's willingness to pay a determined price that dictates strategy. That is, how much does the market want to pay for an industrial medicine program? Does the market want the package of services delivered at a bundled or an unbundled price? How price-sensitive is the buyer? The difference between marketing and finance with regard to price is the difference between the floor and the ceiling.

In an internal perspective, the administrator or the chief financial officer is always concerned about cost and overhead. This is the floor. Pricing below this level leads to a loss. From a marketing perspective, the focus of concern is external, on the ceiling. How high would the market go for a particular service if it saw a value added to it? The difference between the ceiling and the floor represents the margin.

To a large extent, changes in the computer industry reflect the difficulty of premium pricing in health care. Thirty years ago, as an emerging industry, computer companies such as IBM followed a premium pricing strategy. For a new product with a lot of risk for the buyer, the value added to an IBM computer was the brand name of the organization. IBM was the industry standard. Early buyers of computers can remember the term IBM-compatible as the risk factor when one of these name brand alternatives wasn't purchased. Now, however, the products of the computer industry have become commodity goods. It is difficult to premium price a commodity product. IBM, along with manufacturers of other well-known brand names, has seen a precipitate decline in its margins, because consumers are no longer willing to pay a premium. The value added of the brand name is gone.

In health care, the pricing challenge is the same. Ideally, an organization would always prefer to price high. A larger margin is more profitable and allows more room for error. As health care moves to more of a commodity position, however, obtaining a price differential from the buyer is increasingly difficult.

In developing a pricing decision for a service, an important financial concern is break-even analysis. The formula used to calculate a break-even point, the point at which revenue exactly covers fixed and variable costs is:

Break-Even Point = Fixed Cost/(Price - Variable Cost)

The break-even formula also plays an important role in marketing strategy in that it conveys the hurdle rate, which an organization must achieve competitively to cover its costs, when this amount is related to market share. Specifically, there are three elements to the formula: fixed costs, price, and variable costs. Managerially, one might assume that fixed costs are easily quantified, whether it be to build an outpatient surgery center or roll out a new health fitness program for executives in which space must be redesigned, equipment purchased, and personnel hired. The more interesting parts of the formula are price and variable costs. These two aspects of break-even are judgmental—that is, these variables depend on the organization's strategy.

A major issue is whether costs should be viewed as fixed or variable. For example, in rolling out a new service, advertising is often viewed as a necessary budget item. From a marketing person's perspective, then, advertising should be viewed as a fixed cost of the project (i.e., the new service roll-out). However, marketing expenses such as advertising are often considered discretionary items and are not calculated within the fixed cost component of a break-even point. This approach provides an unrealistic estimate of the costs of breaking even in a new project decision.

The amount of sales (or revenue) needed to reach the break-even point can be decreased by increasing the price or by reducing the fixed costs, but the realities of the market must come into play. For example, a health care organization might try to price high as mentioned previously to reduce break-even requirements. The reality check, however, is whether the market will accept the price. Or, the organization could try to reduce variable costs, such as advertising for the new program. The concern here is whether a low-cost strategy will help get market acceptance.

In either case, the break-even formula is an important tool to consider the sensitivity of strategies around price and variable costs (salespeople, promotion, etc.) when tied to market share. It is the representation of the cost of break-even relative to the size of the market that indicates the challenge and inherent risk in the new service rollout. That is, an organization, in developing its marketing strategy, never wants to calculate a single break-even point. Rather, several alternative break-even points that relate to different options regarding price and variable costs should be calculated. These break-even points should then be converted to indicate what market shares are required to meet them. This insight provides some perspective on the sensitivity of marketing strategy to marketplace realities.

In marketing, pricing is also a consideration in positioning the product or service in customers' minds.[10] An organization must decide whether it prefers the price to be high or low relative to the competition and whether price will play an active or a passive part in the positioning of the service. In an active pricing strategy, price is a dominant part of positioning the product or service, and it is prominently displayed in communications. In a passive strategy, attributes other than price are focused on in communication of value to the customer.

Figure 5, below, shows the four quadrants with regard to price positioning. In the high price/active position, the organization makes no excuses that the product costs more. This was the long-standing claim of Curtis Mathes television sets when the company touted "the most expensive television set that money can buy." This position is often used by organizations in which the objective quality of the product is hard to discern or evaluate. Price then becomes a cue for quality.

Figure 5. Price Positioning Matrix

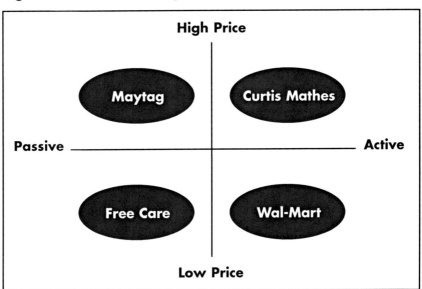

In the low price/active position, Wal-Mart proudly shows advertisements that highlight that its prices are falling daily. This position is being staked out by some Medicare HMO plans. In the passive price position, one could be like Maytag. The company does not focus on the fact that it is a premium priced product, but rather touts the reliability of its appliances. This position is one many health care organizations strive to achieve by highlighting their unique areas of clinical expertise or the level of clinical quality that they are perceived as delivering.

The final price position may be viewed in some ways as an odd alternative, in that the organization has a low price but does not talk about it. In fact, this is a position taken by many hospitals obligated to provide free care. These institutions, however, would never solicit such business. To some extent, the sliding scale pricing strategy of Community Health Centers sponsored by the U.S. Public Health Service uses the low price/ passive position.

Place: Getting the Service

The third component of marketing strategy is place, or distribution. In the traditional product setting, it involves all the decisions of moving a product from producer to consumer. In developing marketing strategies around this component, the organization is concerned with where a service is offered, what hours it might be available, and how it will be accessed. In health care, place or distribution issues focus on decisions regarding the flow of patients through the system. Figure 6, page 69, shows several alternative patient flows through the system, in marketing called the channel of distribution. As can be seen in column A, the simplest flow of patients is to the primary care doctor. As one moves from B through D, other intermediaries often intervene, be they specialists, hospitals, tertiary hospitals, or managed care organizations.

In terms of dealing with patient flow, the goal is to always control this channel of distribution. Two common strategies, referred to as push and pull, are often used in marketing. In a push strategy, the organization develops an approach to work through the intermediaries in the channel. For example, in channel C, the hospital wants to get patients from physicians. Often, these intermediaries, the doctors, have privileges at more than one hospital. One approach might consist of developing a medical office building and giving discounted rent to the doctors. In this way, the physician located next to a particular hospital might encourage patients to be admitted to that facility. Another approach, less cost intensive, might consist of programs to make doctors feel positively toward a particular facility. Weekend retreats, valet parking for physicians, and good lunches in the doctors' lounge are all relatively low-cost ways of encouraging intermediaries in the channel to direct patient flow.

Figure 6. Alternative Patient Flows

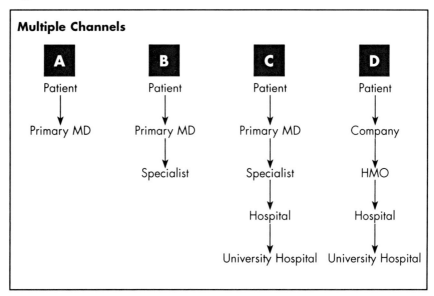

Multiple Channels

A	B	C	D
Patient	Patient	Patient	Patient
↓	↓	↓	↓
Primary MD	Primary MD	Primary MD	Company
	↓	↓	↓
	Specialist	Specialist	HMO
		↓	↓
		Hospital	Hospital
		↓	↓
		University Hospital	University Hospital

The alternative to push approaches is pull strategies. In a pull strategy, the organization bypasses the intermediaries and goes directly to the user, in this case the patient. An HMO, for example, occasionally faces resistance when trying to have its plan offered in a particular company. If the company (figure 6, column D) does not offer the HMO, employees can never access the plan. In this case, the intermediary must be bypassed. The HMO might run an advertisement that says, "If your company does not offer the XYZ HMO, you cannot pick one of the better plans available. Ask your boss why not?" The goal of such an approach is to encourage potential patients to approach the company and demand that the plan be offered. A similar pull strategy is being seen by many hospitals that advertise a particular center of excellence. The purpose is to get the patient to ask the doctor about being admitted to that institution if the problem is relevant. Or, if the doctor does not have privileges at the facility, the patient can bypass the intermediary and go directly to the facility. In order for a pull strategy to work effectively, the organization or service must have very strong brand name recognition. Mayo, for example, can benefit from a pull strategy. A patient told of a major problem might say, "I'm not staying locally. I'm going to the Mayo Clinic." In essence, the reputation of the Mayo Clinic pulls patients around the local physician and specialty referral network.

Pharmaceutical companies have been most aggressive in their use of a pull strategy. The direct marketing to consumers of prescription drugs has become commonplace as these companies became restricted in the type of incentive programs they could use in trying to direct physicians to prescribe their particular product. The dramatic rise in Internet use has resulted in a new distribution channel for services, supplies, pharmaceuticals, and even diagnosis of patient illnesses.

In reality, most organizations use a combination of push and pull strategies to control the channel of distribution. It is essential in the development of marketing strategy to identify the intermediaries in the channel and to develop programs to control the flow of patients.

Promotion

The final element of marketing strategy is promotion. The promotional mix consists of four approaches: public relations, advertising, personal selling, and sales promotions.

In health care, reliance has traditionally been placed on public relations. Public relations can be defined as any non-directly paid presentation or activity for an organization. Public relations activities consist of working with the media for the placement of favorable stories about health care facilities or of sponsoring community programs to create a favorable image of the group within the community. Health fairs, fun runs, and free blood pressure screenings are all common activities that are designed to create a favorable impression.

A major function of public relations is to work to have favorable stories placed in the media about the health care group. Because the attention paid by the media is not directly paid for, a favorable story reported in the press about a doctor, a hospital, or an HMO is of great value. Most people view these stories as having a great deal of credibility. They are viewed differently from an advertisement. Yet, it is in trying to obtain favorable press that the weakness of this approach is revealed. It is the rare physician who has not been interviewed by the media at some length. As most readers of this book can attest, reading an article in which you were interviewed often leads to a reaction such as, "I didn't say that." Because publicity is a function of the media deciding to run the story, there is little control over the message. If the health care organization tries to get the story repeated on a second day, it is unlikely to be successful, because the media no longer view the story as newsworthy. It is because of these limitations that most health care organizations have turned to advertising.

Advertising can be defined as a directly paid form of presentation of a service, product, or organization. Because a health care organization pays the media to run its advertisement, the organization has control over several important elements. The health care organization can control to whom the message is sent, when the message is sent, how often the message is sent, and how the message is sent. The health care provider can decide what newspaper is best, what day of the week the ad should run, how large the ad should be, and how frequently the message should be told. None of these elements can be controlled in a story generated through public relations activities. A major limitation of advertising relative to public relations, however, involves credibility. Consumers understand an advertisement is a form of self-promotion and often process the information more critically.

While the purpose of this chapter is not to explain all the components of creating a successful advertising program, it is important to outline a few key ingredients. A well-run advertising campaign begins with a definition of the target audience. The organization should have a fairly well-defined profile of whom it wants to attract. This aspect was discussed earlier in this chapter and underscores the importance of the organization's clearly defining the target market. In this way, appropriate media can be selected to reach the target audience. Second, a well-run advertising campaign is centered on advertisements that are pre-tested with the intended audience. A major difference to date between many of the advertisements developed in health care and those of more traditional companies has been the lack of pre-testing. Often, in health care organizations, an advertisement is developed internally and then placed with the media. The doctors in the group often review the ad and give approval or suggest some minor changes. In a well-run advertising campaign, the pretest should be conducted with a sample of people for whom the ad is intended. Do these people like the ad? Do they understand what is being said? Is there any additional information that they would like to see in the ad? Finally, in a well-run ad campaign, there is a measurable set of objectives that guide the copy and the media strategy of the campaign.

The third component of promotional strategy is the use of personal selling. Traditionally, salespeople were rare in health care organizations other than HMOs, which had representatives who presented the respective plans within a company. Increasingly, however, the use of personal sales forces for contact with intermediaries in the channel of distribution has grown. Hospitals have used sales representatives to contact physicians; radiology departments have used salespeople to contact referral sources; and adolescent chemical dependency programs have salespeople contacting judges, social workers, and probation officers.[11]

Salespeople can perform multiple roles.[12] The common role is selling or obtaining new business, but salespeople are also useful in conducting field research on the competition or on prospective user needs. Salespeople also play an important missionary role of maintaining goodwill and of dealing with any user complaints or problems. For medical organizations that depend on referrals, this last role is particularly valuable.

The final component of promotional strategy involves the use of sales promotions, the common form being coupons. While a regular strategy for most consumer goods marketers, coupons have infrequently been used in health care. Some reported uses have been the offering of a free health screen for first-time users of a new service, or a small price reduction on the first office visit of a new patient. To a large extent, the value of sales promotions is the ability to track the response to an advertisement. Coupons allow the organization to track whether individuals are reading an ad and finding the offer of sufficient interest to act. In general, the response rate to direct mail coupons is one and one-half to three percent.

Marketing in the Digital Age

The most significant advance in business and marketing may well be the Internet. The explosion of Web-related sites for consumers to access databases, for business-to-business commerce, and for the growing sophistication of marketing strategy is dramatic.[13]

Few aspects of marketing are not touched by this technological revolution. Patients are being directly affected by the ever-increasing use of the Web for second opinions, and results have begun to be reported. For example, several Harvard teaching hospitals have begun offering second opinions and report changing the treatment plans for 90 percent of those patients.[14] And, some organizations, such as the Cancer Center at Baptist Medical Center in Winston Salem, North Carolina, have developed a portal for patients to set up appointments directly (www.wfubmc.edu/hoc/appointment.html). Finally, databases now available on-line will dramatically affect the marketing landscape for organizations. Rating groups such as Leapfrog allow a link to review their ratings of hospitals, physicians, and nursing homes (www.healthgrades.com). In a business-to-business context, one can view the Web sites of organizations such as the Mayo Clinic (www.mayoclinic.org) that have forms to refer a patient to the Clinic.

Finally, the Web has also resulted in significant changes in terms of promotional strategy. While measurement of their effectiveness is being developed, pop-up advertisements are increasingly common. While the demise of the dotcoms slowed the optimistic growth forecasts of on-line advertising, industry observers still believe it will be a major force in promotional strategy.[15,16]

Summary

Marketing is a process that focuses on the buyers of a service. Essential to the development of any effective marketing strategy is the need to understand buyers' requirements and demands. Contrary to traditional health care planning, which is motivated by the requirements of those internal to the organization, marketing is an external-to-internal approach. After fully understanding buyers' requirements, the organization develops a strategy based on the four components of the marketing mix: product, price, place, and promotion.

References

1. For a comprehensive perspective on the nature of marketing and the role of consumer input, see Kerin, and others. *Marketing*, Seventh Edition. Homewood, Ill.: Richard D. Irwin, Inc., 2003, chap. 1.

2. A detailed discussion of secondary data sources in health care is provided in Hillestad, S., and Berkowitz, E. *Health Care Marketing Plans: From Strategy to Action,* Second Edition. Rockville, Md.: Aspen Publishers, 1991, pp. 90-96.

3. Kotler, P., and Armstrong, G. *Principles of Marketing.* Upper Saddle River, N.J.: Prentice Hall, 2004.

4. A useful reference on focus groups is Kreuger, R. *Focus Groups: A Practical Guide for Applied Research.* Newbury Park, Calif.: Sage Press, 1988.

5. A useful article to see the application of telephone interviewing is Gombeski, W., and others. "Overnight Assessment of Marketing Crises." *Journal of Health Care Marketing* 11(1):51-4, March 1991.

6. Porter, M. *Competitive Advantage: Creating and Sustaining Superior Performance.* New York, N.Y.: Free Press, 1985.

7. Berkowitz, E., and others. *Marketing.* New York, N.Y.: McGraw Hill, 2000, chap. 10.

8. Duboff, R. "Marketing to Maximize Profitability." *Journal of Business Strategy* 13(6):10-3, Nov.-Dec. 1992.

9. Meredith, G., Schewe, C., and Karlovich, J. *Defining Markets, Defining Moments.* New York, N.Y.: Hungry Minds Press, 2002.

10. Tellis, G. "Creative Pricing Strategies for Medical Services." *Journal of Medical Practice Management* 3(2):120-4, Fall 1987.

11. Bates, B., and McSurley, H. "The Sales Function in Radiology Departments." *Administrative Radiology* 8(9):16-9, Sept. 1989.

12. Mack, K., and Newbold, P. *Health Care Sales.* San Francisco, Calif.: Jossey-Bass Publishers, 1991, chap. 1.

13. Kotler, P., and Armstrong, G., *op. cit.,* chap. 3.

14. Kowalczyk, L. "Second Opinions Given Online Help Patients, Study Says."

Boston Globe, March 29, 2003, p. D2

15. Noerton, R. "The Bright Future of Web Advertising." *E-company Now,* June 2001, pp. 55-60.

16. Noerton, R. "Summit Participants Agree Online Poised for Growth." *Advertising Age,* April, 1, 2002, p. C6

Eric N. Berkowitz, PhD is Associate Dean, Professional Programs and Professor of Marketing, University of Massachusetts, Amherst.

Chapter 5

Making the Most of Medical Management

by Sandra L. Gill, PhD

Introduction

Physicians must manage or be managed—in their clinical practice, their groups, the medical staff, hospital and health care organization. This chapter identifies key skills for physician managers to become more successful in personal, group and organizational efforts.

Effective management is about others.

Effective physician managers will need a wealth of personal skills to cope with the vortex of competing demands upon them. A healthy dose of genuine self-esteem, a clear set of personal core values, personal will and physical endurance, appreciation for one's limits and power, a sense of perspective and sense of humor will all be drawn upon daily.

Much of modern management cultivates a sense of the leader and manager as an individual hero. Indeed, most leaders need to make heroic efforts to achieve great ends during their tenure. But recent research differentiates the direction of ego and self interest—"away from themselves and into the larger goal of building a great company."[1] Jim Collins identifies a five level hierarchy where highly capable individuals are *at the bottom*. It's the combination of humility + will, a kind of resolve and selflessness, a tenacity to make really tough decisions to get results for the greater good of the organization. The difference, says Collins, is simple—for some people, work is all about what they *get*—fame, fortune, adulation, power vs. what they *build*, create and contribute. Level 5 leaders are "more plow horse than show horse." Their ego is directed to building for others, for a legacy larger than themselves.

Briefly, Collins' 2001 model captures the remaining four levels of his hierarchy as follows. Level 1 are Highly Capable Individuals, who are productive, talented, skillful and have good work habits. Level 2 are Contributing Team Members, contributing their individual talents to the group, working effectively in group settings. Level 3 are Competent Managers, who can organize resources and pursue predetermined objectives. Level 4 are Effective Leaders, who catalyze commitment and stimulate higher performance standards in pursuit of a compelling vision.

The two sides of Collins' Level 5 leaders use their professional will to help create exceptional results, focused with unwavering commitment to long term, enduring goals, and accepting responsibility instead of seeking to blame. Their humility avoids boasting, using their personal high standards to motivate by example, groom successors and apportion credit to others. Indeed, it's rare in most organizations, but not rare in our society. The critical factor is ego—for self or others. Self-oriented leaders can certainly obtain results, but usually not for very long since its for personal benefit. Level 5 leaders transform those around them—others merely transact with people around them, often in a highly effective but not generative fashion. Level 5 leaders attract a team with similar values, and then build the path to greatness. The good to great management teams will debate vigorously for the best answers, and then support decisions, beyond individual or parochial interests.

Endurance and energy are essential

In my work with thousands of physicians over 20 years, I've used a variety of assessment instruments, among them the Myers-Briggs Type Indicator (MBTI).[2]

This very popular assessment reveals personal preferences in the direction of one's mental energy, the kinds of perception and judgment one prefers, and general orientation or approach to the world. The four mental processes of Sensing, Intuition, Thinking, and Feeling, along with one's tendency to focus on one's inner (introverted) or outer (extraverted) world reveal a familiar four letter code.[3]

In dozens of workshops with hundreds of physician leaders, I have found more Introversion than Extraversion, indicating that physicians' primary source of mental energy comes from within. Physicians also ranked highly on Sensing as a way to gather information, even when they preferred Intuition, and predominantly preferred to use Thinking over Feeling as a decision-making strategy. They predominantly preferred to manage their outer worlds as decision-makers, using Judging over the information-gathering fashion indicated by Perceiving.[4] Thus, while physicians report-ed the use of every dimension, and while there are specialty differences— more intuition among psychiatrists, more sensing among surgeons, for example— the predominant pattern among physician leaders was for introversion (I); sensing (S), thinking (T) and judging (J).

This "ISTJ" pattern , while stereotypical, offers considerable insight for medical managers.

Introversion and Extraversion—Your source of mental energy

Medical management is essentially relational—almost constant interac-tion with groups and teams, and almost no privacy. Introverts draw their mental energy from within, and constant interaction in larger groups may leave highly introverted persons feeling drained. Physicians with a high preference for introversion reported this exhausting aspect in their leadership roles, saying how they coveted the quiet, intimate interaction with a patient in the exam room, if they continued practice as a medical manager. Introverts may even be so reflective and succinct that they invite second guessing—and it's almost always negative:

"She didn't say she liked it, in fact she hardly said anything at all;" "every-one smiled except Dr. _____ so I guess he didn't like it.", etc.

While introverts rejected the seemingly overt, attention-getting expres-siveness of highly extraverted persons, they almost always admired the verbal fluency, congruent verbal and non-verbal communication and overt energy their extraverted colleagues brought to leadership roles. Introverted leaders generally need to express themselves more often than they consider necessary. They may need to practice positive feedback, frequent smiling and non-verbal affirmation, and make a habit to reply more quickly than they would prefer. Most of all, however, introverted leaders will have to find sufficient "space" to restore their depleted ener-gies from constant interaction. Tired people make mistakes, so it's essen-tial to respect your source of mental energy—from within, for more intro-verted persons, and through interaction for more extraverted people.

Physicians suggested many resources for restoring their energies: playing classical music in their office background taking a brisk walk, scheduling appointments for work time and time alone, working before or after staff were present using e-mail and voice mail as a substitute for non-essential meetings, and scheduling time for exercise—alone or with headphones! In short, the interactive demands in virtually every medical management role seriously affected the more highly introverted physicians, so respecting one's source of energy became an essential daily practice.

Sensing and Intuition—Ways of Perceiving

Medical managers must also cope with numerous organizational decisions that lack sufficient supporting facts. The relentless pressures in our competitive marketplace limit time and resources for thorough analysis, time after time. While "intuitives' may enjoy this novelty and complexity, high "sensors" may reject such imperfection, wanting verification and more tangible evidence. Physicians routinely reported the impact of scientific, medical training on their highly developed sensing, to the point where intuition was even repressed. Yet, in management, many issues require the use of intuition for early warning, or creative re-combinations of limited resources to intractable, complex problems.

Thinking and Feeling—Frameworks for Decision-Making

The popularity of Emotional Intelligence (EI)[5,6] and its focus on the value of emotional self awareness, empathy and relational skills has invigorated contemporary leadership and management. While physicians reported the predominant reliance on "hard, cold reason" throughout their medical training, they also expressed keen training in "bedside manner." Goleman's work on EI posits that the personal competencies of self awareness, self regulation, self-motivation, along with the social competencies of empathy and social awareness will differentiate effective from highly effective leaders.[7]

Indeed, physicians expressed the value of the "softer" skills from more "feeling oriented" persons, who expressed empathy, appreciation of others and quest for harmony versus conflict.

The high rate of conflict among physicians, while rationalized as part of the rigor to sustain scientific, evidence based action, also has high costs. The natural skepticism of "thinkers," can be raised to an unnatural level of constant criticism as a result of medical training—and this will be disastrous for medical managers. Effective managers must find and use gentle, more respectful phrases that can sustain relationships while also elevating inquiry. For example, "Help me understand;" "That's different from my personal experience;" "I respectfully disagree."

Judging vs. Perceiving—Orientation to the World

A preference for judging, especially used in the outer world, connotes your preference for either Thinking or Feeling in decision making. Thinking Judgers (TJ), as most physicians reported themselves, seek logical analyses, are comfortable with questions and often remain skeptical. Feeling Judgers, in contrast, may seek harmony and express empathy, and have very firm feelings of what's "right"—or wrong—in actions toward others. Thinking judging can appear to be highly critical—even cruel. While skepticism may be well-intended, i.e., to sustain valid, rigorous solutions, it can easily become a raging conflict.

Perceiving is a means of managing one's outer world, just as Judging is. Those who manage by perceiving enjoy sponteneity, novelty, variety and will want to improvise--quite in contrast to the "judgers" who prefer order, structure and methodical approaches. Perceivers may be criticized for their more casual, emergent and open-ended approach, where they often wish to examine yet one more possibility. Yet this flexibility is invaluable in many situations. Perceivers are likely to adapt rather than resist, create rather than debate, and advance rather than argue over something that has been changed.

Conflict Resolution—A Core Competency

Beyond these personal phrases and professional commitment to healthy relationships, physician managers must learn a variety of protocols for resolving conflict.[8] Complex organizations and creative people produce conflict, yet many physicians reported enormous aversion to dealing with conflict.

Most of us employ a variety of approaches to dealing with conflict—avoidance, accommodation, agreement or compliance, and competition or argumentation.[9] Managers are inherently in the middle of things, perhaps significantly different from the previous role of the physician in the clinical setting. Thus, effective conflict management skills become crucial. The challenge for medical managers is to manage the conflict rather than try to eliminate it.[10]

Reframing the conflict can transform the outcome, from a competitive, right wrong, win-lose context to a more insightful difference of perspective. By adopting an "abundance mentality" where all can be right vs. win-lose, along with respectful yet honest communication, people can move from conflict to collaboration or even synergy. As Sitting Bull once said, "Offer your opponent the peace pipe first." When you change, others can change. Synergy emerges only from collaboration, not competition.

Competition may well be appropriate, such as when time is short and you are sure you are correct, or when the other party would take unfair advantage of you. But being "right" may be wrong, when the conflict is trivial, or when good relationships really matter. Medical managers must become astute assessors of the conflict situation, and be skilled in a repertoire of conflict resolution protocols. For example, *Getting to Yes*[11] and *Difficult Conversations*[12] emphasize the importance of "being hard on the issue" but "soft on the people." Like most of medical practice, skills in conflict resolution can be enhanced through training and practice. Numerous assessment tools are available to identify one's conflict management style and recognize its strengths and weaknesses, such as the Thomas-Kilmann Conflict Mode Instrument.[13] Engaging in role reversal with a trustworthy fellow executive, where each take's on the other's perspective and spontaneously play out attempts to resolve conflict, can provide enormous insight, calm feelings of anger and frustration and provide a safe practice opportunity.

Relationships, almost always outlast solutions, so building constructive relationships to revise current solutions and resolve future conflicts, inevitable in complex organizations, is an essential competency.

Team Building

Most physicians bring vast experience in the high performance of critical care teams. Day to day medical management, however, often lacks the urgent conditions under which talented individuals suppress their personal differences to "save" a patient. Indeed, the physician manager's authority may be challenged, rather than respected, in many events. Demands may be for very good team performance, rather than heroic efforts appropriate in critical care. Effective medical managers have a repertoire of team building skills to move groups to high performing teams.

Key competencies for being a team leader include personal flexibility; effective communication; and skills in team building, conflict management, and change management.[14] Many physicians already have experience in quality improvement approaches to team facilitation, including effective meeting design and facilitation; project management and creativity techniques.

A newer tool, called Appreciative Inquiry (AI), builds on success, using a whole system model, in contrast to the TQM tools that focus on problem identification or weaknesses, usually in a defined service unit. Appreciative Inquiry incorporates three principles. (1) people respond to positive knowledge; (2) the shared vision of the future and process for developing this vision create the energy to drive change, and (3) that affirmation and envisioning goals increases the likelihood of transforming goals into reality.[15] By building on four primary questions, a transformational approach to organizational change can be facilitated. AI begins with appreciating, by discovering the best of what is, the dreams about what might be, moving to the design of an ideal approach, and then sustaining the team's dream through learning, empowerment, adjustments and improvising. AI recognizes that whole system change emerges from whole system inquiry, blending shared efforts into what must change to achieve a desired future.[16]

Other large and whole system facilitation techniques also incorporate visualization, story telling and metaphors to inspire meaningful results.[17,18] For example, stories about when one felt "most like a leader," "making a significant difference," or "being at your best" invoke highly inspirational incidents that can serve as models for the whole organization. One health system recently engaged a storyteller to describe the patient care experience as a mother of an asthmatic child, comparing its current system with its envisioned, clinically integrated patient care model.[19]

In summary, contemporary medical managers must augment medical training and experience with a repertoire of personal and team building skills. Personal attributes and decision-making preferences that may have been rewarded in clinical practice will be challenged in the larger group settings of complex organizations. Reliance on professional expertise, while necessary, is not sufficient. Skill and practice in small group and whole system change management are solid investments for today's medical manager.

References

1. Collins, J. *Good to Great: Why Some Companies Make the Leap and Others Don't.* New York: Harper, 2001, p. 21.

2. Myers-Briggs Type Indicator. Palo Alto, CA: CPP, Inc.

3. Pearman, Roger R. *An Introduction to Type and Emotional Intelligence: Pathways to Performance.* Palo Alto, CA: CPP, Inc., 2002.

4. Additional data on physicians and many other professions may be found in M.H. McCauley's (1978) Application of Myers-Briggs Type Indicator to medicine and other health professions, Monograph I, Contract No. 231-76-0051, Health Resources Administration, DHEW, and from the CAPT-MBTI Atlas, Center for the Application of Psychological Type, Gainesville, Florida.

5. Goleman, Daniel. *What Makes a Leader?* Cambridge, MA: Harvard Business School Press, 1999.

6. Druskat, V. U. and S. B. Wolff. *Building the Emotional Intelligence of Groups.* Cambridge, MA: Harvard Business School. March, 2001, pp. 81-90. Product #620X.

7. Goleman, D. *Working with Emotional Intelligence.* New York: Bantam Books, 1998.

8. Cohn, Kenneth H., M.D., and Peetz, Michael E. M.D. "Surgeon Frustration: Contemporary Problems, Practical Solutions." May 7, 2003 presentation to Maine Health System.

9. Thomas-Kilmann Conflict Mode Instrument, Palo Alto, CA: Consulting Psychologists Press, Inc.

10. Aldag, R. and L. Kuzuhara. *Organizational Behavior and Management: An Integrated Skills Approach.* Cincinnati, Ohio: South-Western Thomson, 2002, p. 466.

11. Fisher, R. William Ury, and Bruce Patton. *Getting to Yes: Negotiating Agreement Without Giving In.* New York: Penguin Books, 1991.

12. Stone, Douglas, Bruce Patton and Sheila Heen. *Difficult Conversations: How to discuss what matters most.* New York: Penguin, 1999.

13 Thomas-Kilmann Conflict Mode Instrument, Palo Alto, CA: Consulting Psychologists Press, Inc.

14. Gill, Sandra L. An Exploration of Physician Leadership Roles and Related Competencies Across Health Care Market Stages. Unpublished dissertation. The Fielding Graduate Institute, Santa Barbara, CA, 1998.

15. Johnson, G., and Leavitt, W. "Transforming organizations through an appreciative inquiry." *Public Personnel Management* 30 (1) 129-135, 2001.

16. Cooperrider, David. *Appreciative Inquiry: Rethinking Human Organization Toward a Positive Theory of Change.* Champaign, IL: Stipes Publishing, 2000.

17. Bunker, B., and Alban, B. *Large Group Interventions: Engaging the Whole System for Rapid Change.* San Francisco, CA: Jossey-Bass, 1997.

18. Laszlo, C. & Laugel, J.F. *Large-Scale Organizational Change: An Executives Guide.* Woburn, MA: Butterworth-Heinemann, 2000.

19. Gawlik, G., M.D. Central DuPage Health, Winfield, Illinois.

Sandra L. Gill, PhD, is Dean, College of Business and Associate Professor of Business, Benedictine University, Lisle, Illinois. For over 30 years, Dr. Gill has served as on-site faculty with the American College of Physician Executives, and has completed more than 1,000 health care consulting engagements as President of Physician Management Resources, Inc. Dr. Gill may be contacted at sgill@ben.edu.

Chapter 6

Improving the Quality of Medical Care

by Harry L. Leider, MD, MBA, FACPE
and David B. Nash, MD, MBA, FACPE

Although leaders in medicine have long sought to improve the quality of medical care, it is only recently that the need to improve care has become an imperative for the medical profession and for our populace. This chapter will address three fundamental issues: why the need to improve quality of care is more important than in the past, why the overall quality of medical care is sub-optimal, and how we can improve quality of medical care.

Why the Need to Improve Quality of Medical Care Is Growing in Importance

Researchers and academicians in health care have long known that quality of care can be improved. However several events and factors over the past decade made this a major issue for our nation. In the mid-1990s, managed care grew rapidly and contributed to bringing down the rampant medical cost inflation of the late 1980s and early 1990s. However, the tactics used by managed care organizations, such as requiring patients to have referrals from their primary care doctors to see specialists and aggressive utilization management practices caused many patients to begin to question the quality of care they received and, in many cases, lessened the historic strong bonds of trust between patients and their doctors.

Superimposed on this environment of distrust was a seminal report released in 1999 by the Institute of Medicine.[1] This report estimated that between 44,000 and 98,000 patients die in hospitals each year because of medical errors. The report put this in perspective by stating that, even at the lower figure, the deaths due to error exceed deaths due to automobile accidents, breast cancer, and AIDS. These figures were widely reported in the popular press, as were subsequent cases of serious medical errors.

A second report by the Institute of Medicine went further and stated: "The U.S. health care delivery system does not provide consistent, high-quality medical care to all people. Americans should be able to count on receiving care that meets their needs and is based on the best scientific knowledge—yet there is strong evidence that this is frequently not the case. Health care harms patients too frequently and routinely fails to deliver its potential benefits. Indeed, between the health care that we now have and the health care that we could have lies not just a gap, but a chasm...."[2]

In essence, this report stated that, despite having the best acute care services in the world, the overall U.S. heath care system is essentially broken and fails to deliver consistent quality, especially for patients with chronic illnesses. The report continues by laying out some principles and next steps for improving quality and beginning to "cross the quality chasm."

At the same time these reports were released, another powerful trend reinforced the importance of improving quality. Beginning in the late 1990s, health care cost inflation rapidly increased. By 2001, on average, employers experienced annual health insurance premium increases of more than 10 percent, and this rate of cost inflation has continued.[3] This increased burden led many employers to actively question the quality of the care and services provided to their employees. Coalitions of large employers, such as the Washington Business Group on Health, the Pacific Business Group on Health, and the Leapfrog Group, created and launched initiatives directed at holding managed care organizations, hospitals, and physicians more accountable for the quality of care provided to their beneficiaries.[4-6]

Finally, in reaction to the rapid increases in their health care costs, most employers passed on some of them through a variety of mechanisms, including higher employee premium contributions, deductibles, co-payments for physicians' visits, and co-payments for drugs. This strategy of shifting some of the costs to patients while providing them with tools and information to make good decisions is often labeled "consumerism."[7] As a result of having to bear more of the financial burden for their medical care, patients are much more actively questioning the quality of the care and services they receive. The growing availability of health care information on the Internet has accelerated this trend. In summary, the dissemination of major reports highlighting major problems with quality of care, increasing activism by employers, and the growing role of the patient/consumer have together created an environment in which all stakeholders are much more concerned with medical care quality. The public and those who pay for medical care are now interested in knowing whether they are getting a good value for their health care dollars.

Why Quality of Medical Care Is Sub-Optimal

Although there have been many attempts to define quality, there is no single comprehensive definition of medical quality, most likely because quality encompasses several different elements and aspects of care. Avedis Donabedian, often referred to as the founder of health care quality assurance, extensively reviewed and categorized the various aspects of medical quality.[8] The major components he described are effectiveness, efficiency, optimality, and acceptability of medical care.

Quality is often viewed as having two broad dimensions: the technical aspects of care and the interpersonal aspects of care.[9] Technical quality relates to how well patients are diagnosed and treated, while interpersonal quality depends on how well the personal needs of patients are met. Other definitions of quality incorporate evaluations of patient preferences and considerations for the cost of care.

- "Quality is the degree to which the process of care increases the probability of outcomes desired by patients and decreases the probability of undesired outcomes, given the state of medical knowledge."[10]
- "Quality health care consists of necessary medical processes that result in cure, significant measured improvement in the patient's condition, alleviation of pain or other desired outcomes, and provides real value for the dollars spent."[11]

Newer research confirms that we now have the tools to classify most quality-related problems as underuse, overuse, or misuse and that large numbers of Americans are harmed as a direct result of these issues.[12]

Regardless of which definition we choose, several underlying factors contribute to our "quality problem." These include lack of agreement on how to measure quality (as discussed above), variation in clinical practice, rapidly changing clinical knowledge, overemphasis on care for the acute ill (vs. care for the chronically ill), lack of collaboration among health care professionals, poorly aligned incentives, and insufficient technology supports. In addition, the delivery of medical care is a complicated process that involves many people (not just physicians) and many "steps." We will discuss this last issue in more detail later in the chapter, however at this point it is important to recognize that the inherent complexity of health care processes is a major driver of sub-optimal quality.

A growing body of research demonstrates the existence of wide variations in clinical practices. Research conducted by Wennberg[13-15] revealed the significance of variations in the rate of different medical and surgical procedures within small geographic areas. These variations could not be explained by differences in patients' medical conditions and did not correspond to differences in health outcome. Therefore they are attributable to differences in physician practice styles.[13] This research suggests that patients in some geographical areas may receive unnecessary care, while others may not receive needed care.

Additional studies conducted by researchers at the RAND Corporation revealed that as much as one-third of medical care may be unnecessary or of little benefit.[16-17] These results raised questions as to the "best" or "most effective" treatment for some medical conditions and contributed to concerns about the value and the quality of medical interventions. Inappropriate care in the form of under- or overutilization of services highlighted a great need to measure the appropriateness and the outcomes of various medical interventions.[18]

Rapidly changing clinical knowledge is also a major factor affecting medical quality. Until recently, it was considered poor quality and perhaps malpractice to prescribe a beta-blocker for patients with congestive heart failure. Recent trials have now established beta-blockers as an important component of treatment for heart failure that reduces hospitalizations and mortality.[19,20] Similarly, a recent landmark study concludes that arthroscopy of the knee, a widely used procedure, is not beneficial to the vast majority of patients with osteoarthritis.[21] It is difficult if not impossible for physicians to keep up with all the latest medical knowledge, much less to incorporate this knowledge effectively into their practices.

The previously mentioned IOM report provides a good review of the some of the other issues contributing to poor quality.[2] While we frequently provide superb acute care (e.g., cardiac procedures, trauma services, NICU units, MRI scans), as a nation we have not invested in or organized our health system to provide high-quality, coordinated care to patients with chronic illnesses. Providing care to patients with chronic disease or complex medical problems requires a high degree of coordination among a wide range of health care professionals and stakeholders, including primary care physicians, specialists, home health nurses, case managers, social workers, and mental health professionals, as well as the patient and family caregivers.

In most cases, the dominant fee-for-services and DRG reimbursement models do not encourage physicians and hospitals to focus on and develop processes to coordinate care for the chronically ill. These compensation mechanisms also do not directly compensate providers for investing in technologies (e.g. electronic medical records and physician order entry systems) and the infrastructure that can improve quality of care or facilitate communication among providers. Together these factors led us to the current paradox: we have the most technologically sophisticated medical care in the world, especially with respect to acute services, but, in aggregate, we provide sup-optimal quality of care to our population.

How to Improve Quality of Medical Care

Physicians have long recognized the need to develop and implement new approaches to measure and improve quality. But they have viewed traditional quality assessment efforts as intrusive and largely ineffectual. This opinion developed primarily because these programs relied exclusively on case-by-case inspections of medical records and used quality measures developed with little input from physicians. In addition, while inspecting physician and hospital performance allows quality assurance staff to track problems and look for trends, it detects problems only after they occur and does little to prevent their recurrence. Finally, this traditional approach fails to recognize health care delivery as a series of linked processes requiring the coordinated efforts of many health care professionals. It also does not facilitate systematic analysis and subsequent improvement in patient outcomes.

With respect to measurement of quality, Donabedian established a framework that stresses that quality can be measured not only in terms of the structure and process of care but also in terms of the outcomes of care.[22] Structure is composed of the physical, human, and organizational properties of the setting in which care is provided. These properties include things such as equipment and the number of licensed doctors and nurses on staff. Process consists of the technical aspects of providing care and the procedures used to ensure that patients receive necessary care. For instance, adherence to widely accepted practices and regulatory requirements are measures of process. Outcome encompasses changes in patient health status or satisfaction that can be attributed to the medical care provided. Examples include mortality rates, adverse event rates, and changes in an individual's health-related well-being.

While information about structure and processes of care are related to the probability of obtaining good patient outcomes, they do not necessarily correlate highly with patient outcomes. In the past, health care regulatory agencies concentrated on measuring the structure and process of care, with little attention given to outcomes. More recently, these organizations are also starting to measure and focus on clinical outcomes.

Numerous health services researchers contributed to the growing body of knowledge about how to evaluate and improve the quality of medical care. As new approaches to measuring and managing medical quality continue to evolve, it is likely that techniques will be drawn from several different sources and will be integrated into a comprehensive approach. The developing fields of continuous quality improvement, clinical practice guidelines, outcomes management, and disease management will provide a solid basis for creating successful programs to improve quality.[11]

Continuous Quality Improvement

Continuous quality improvement (CQI), or total quality management (TQM) as it is sometimes referred to in health care, evolved from the manufacturing industry's experience with quality management. Industrial quality experts state that quality means "a continuous effort by all members of the organization to meet the needs and expectations of the customer."[23] Quality management utilizes a number of methods that increase the probability of improving quality. Central to these methods is the use of multidisciplinary teams to identify problems, collection of data and subsequent analysis to understand and correct underlying root causes of problems, and intervention to reduce unwanted complexity and variation in systems through the use of statistical process control theory.[24]

Furthermore, TQM creates an open climate that fosters self-motivation and cooperation, where everyone in the organization shares responsibility for improving quality, not just the leaders. Attempts are made to break down barriers between departments, to improve communication throughout the organization, and to "drive out fear." CQI emphasizes that processes, not individual workers, should be the focus of quality improvement efforts. It is based on a belief that most workers are conscientious and are trying to do a good job, but face a multitude of system problems and complex processes that contribute to poor quality.

By fully analyzing a process and understanding the root causes of variation, workers can develop and implement a plan to improve the process.[25] CQI methods have been used successfully outside health care for a number of years and have resulted in significant improvements in the quality of products and services in fields such as the automotive and semiconductor industries.

Evolution of CQI in Health Care

Application of these quality improvement techniques to health care intrigued many health care leaders, and these approaches have been successful in a number of organizations. One of the initial success stories was the National Demonstration Project on Quality Improvement in Health Care.[26] In 1987, this ambitious one-year project matched 21 well-known health care organizations with experts in the field of industrial quality management. The nationwide experiment demonstrated that CQI techniques could be successfully used in the health care setting.

CQI has continued to gain considerable attention in health care, as is evidenced by the ever-increasing number of presentations at quality improvement conferences and by articles in the literature. A nationwide survey conducted by the American Hospital Association in 1990 reported that 44 percent of all respondents had adopted CQI methods to some degree.[27] In 1992, it was noted that some 1,500 hospitals and health care organizations, as well as the Health Care Financing Administration (now the Centers for Medicare and Medicaid Services), were actively involved in using continuous quality improvement techniques.[28]

Many health care organizations, including payers and providers, learned about CQI and worked on collaborative projects through the Institute for Health Care Improvement.[29] One highly successful project is Idealized Design of Clinical Office Practices (IDCOP). Participants in this collaborative project sought to dramatically improve the efficiency and level of service within the typical outpatient office. Using CQI techniques, the project team created what many now call the "Open-Access Model." A basic component of this model involves holding a majority of appointment slots open each day for "same-day" appointments. For many providers who subsequently adopted this model, the result in terms of patient satisfaction, staff satisfaction, office efficiency, and panel size have been compelling.[30]

Some of the key concepts of CQI are:

- Poor quality usually stems from complex processes or variation within a system and not from individuals' lack of knowledge or skills.
- Because most work is accomplished through process, the focus of CQI is on evaluating and improving processes, not on identifying individuals with bad behavior and trying to change them.
- Quality needs to be built into processes so that poor quality is prevented upstream, not measured by inspection at the end of the line.
- Quality can always be improved. Just meeting the minimum established thresholds for acceptability or compliance does not ensure high quality.
- Quality is based on a thorough understanding of the needs and expectations of customers, both internal and external.
- Decisions are based on facts and scientific measurements, not on presumptions or anecdotal evidence.
- Poor quality is costly and results from unwanted variations and complexity in processes.

Tools and Techniques of CQI

Although a number of CQI models are used in health care, most encompass the following general steps[26] to improve a process or fix a quality problem:

1. Clearly defined goals and objectives for the project are developed.
2. A multidisciplinary project team that understands the process is formed.
3. The team collects data to analyze the process and understand the key steps, variables, and root causes that contribute to quality problems.
4. A plan to improve the process is developed, implemented, and tested.
5. Data are collected and analyzed statistically to track the results of the improvement plan and to measure variation in the process.

This cycle of continuously improving quality begins with identification of priority areas for improvements and then moves on to data collection and analysis. The remaining steps are better known as the "Plan-Do-Check-Act" cycle. Throughout this cycle, cross-functional teams trained in CQI techniques use a variety of data-driven tools to analyze process-related problems, reduce variations in the process, and monitor improvements in the process. If the team using this approach appropriately identifies the underlying root causes of poor quality and makes the necessary changes, waste, rework, complexity, and the associated costs of poor quality can be reduced.[31]

Some of the tools that CQI teams use during the quality improvement cycle include[32]:

- Flowcharts to describe the sequence of steps that occur in a process. They provide a point of common agreement on what the process entails and help the group to focus on areas of redundancy and rework.
- Cause and effect diagrams (e.g., "fishbone" diagrams) to help identify and organize underlying root causes of problems or factors critical to the process.
- Pareto charts (bar graphs) to illustrate the frequency and the impact of various problems in a process and help in the selection of improvement efforts. The Pareto chart is an extension of the Pareto Principle, which states that the majority of problems in a process can be attributed to relatively few factors.
- Histograms and scattergrams to organize and characterize data while relationships among variables are identified.
- Run charts to examine data for trends and patterns that occur over time.

- Control charts to monitor a process for statistical control. Upper and lower statistical "limits" are established to define normal variation from the mean. Points falling outside the control limits represent variations due to special causes.
- Benchmarking to compare the practices of an organization with the practices of leaders in the field. The goal is to identify and learn from the "best practices" and then to adopt those practices.[33]

As CQI has become more widespread, some health care professionals have wondered whether these efforts will replace quality assurance departments altogether. In practice, CQI is often developed and implemented with the help of existing QA programs and personnel. QA staff members often become a valuable resource for training and facilitating the work of cross-functional project teams. Each organization will likely develop its own approach within the context of its quality management program.

Barriers to CQI

Barriers to implementation of CQI in the health care sector have been described in detail by Ziegenfuss.[34] Most of these barriers relate to multiple factors, including; technological, structural, psychosocial, managerial, or cultural issues. Also, a number of organizational barriers may arise because of the complex nature of health care work, inadequate personnel, power conflicts, or concerns for authority over quality improvement programs. One of the most frequently mentioned challenges is difficulty in involving physicians in CQI activities. Reasons cited by physicians for their lack of involvement include lack of time for or commitment to organization-wide activities.[26]

Clinical Guidelines

Clinical pathways or guidelines are used to define the optimal sequence of events and timing for specific medical interventions. The need for guidelines is based on the large degree of variation in clinical practice and on the fact that clinical knowledge is rapidly changing. Guidelines are a tool to reduce variation and disseminate clinical knowledge. They are usually developed through the collaborative efforts of health care professionals to reduce length of stay, delays, and variation in care. They also help to improve communication among physicians, nurses, and other health care professionals.[35]

Despite the widespread development and dissemination of guidelines, physicians frequently still consider guidelines to be "cookbook medicine" and don't adhere to them. Cabana and colleagues reviewed 76 published studies that tried to identify the barriers to guidelines adoption and articulated a "differential diagnosis" for the problem and a framework for improving adherence to guidelines.[36] The main barriers identified in this review included:

- Lack of awareness that a guideline exists
- Lack of familiarity with the details of the guideline
- Lack of agreement with the guideline
- Lack of self-efficacy or inability to follow the guideline
- Lack of outcome expectancy or belief that following the guideline will improve outcomes
- Inertia of previous practice patterns
- External barriers to following the guideline
- Patient-related barriers such as non-compliance

However, many organizations are overcoming these barriers and achieving success using clinical guidelines. For example, San Diego Children's Hospital won the prestigious Codman award for quality in health care by implementing guidelines for 60 procedures and illness and documenting significant improvements in patient care and clinical outcomes.[37]

Creating clinical guidelines can be time-consuming and costly. Therefore, most health care organizations now try to start with "seed" guidelines already created by a professional organization (e.g., the American Heart Association or the National Institutes of Health). Another excellent resource for "seed guidelines" is the U.S. Agency for Healthcare Research and Quality, which hosts a national clearinghouse for guidelines hosted on a website.[38]

Outcomes management combines the use of clinical practice guidelines with the results of outcomes research and focuses on finding out what works from patients' points of view. Outcomes management relies on the use of "standards and guidelines to assist physicians in selecting interventions; it routinely and systematically measures the functioning and well-being of patients; it pools clinical and outcome data on a large scale; and it attempts to analyze and disseminate results from the segment of the database most appropriate to the concerns of each decision maker."[39]

Outcome measures go beyond traditional measures of morbidity and mortality and consider patient satisfaction with the care received, changes in patients' functional abilities, and health-related quality of life. Outcomes management also measures quality from patients' perspectives. While the technical aspects of clinical quality may have been the primary focus of many quality assurance programs, increased attention is now being given to the dimension of quality associated with interpersonal aspects of care.

This dimension considers patient preferences for treatment options, patient-practitioner relationships, and conveniences and courtesies of the medical service provided.[8]

The attention given to this dimension of health care quality is becoming more evident as managed care organizations generate "report cards," with the results of patient ratings for satisfaction with physician office hours, waiting times, and friendliness of physicians and office staff.[40] As competition in health care increases and as providers seek to attract patients to particular health care facilities, this dimension will likely gain more attention and will be used to compare various health care programs.

Using patient satisfaction and outcomes as indicators of quality has led to questions about who should judge the quality of patient outcomes. Health economists suggest that "the ultimate judge of quality and value of a product or service should be the consumer. Thus medical quality can be defined by the nature of the medical outcome as perceived by the patient."[41] Outcomes research will provide information about the care that best reflects the needs and wants of health care consumers. This is entirely consistent with the new emphasis on measuring quality from patients' perspectives and reflects the customer-driven focus of CQI. It is no longer sufficient to measure quality by the traditional "assessment by inspection." Instead, quality must be built into health care processes, and outcomes of care must be measured in an ongoing fashion so that unwanted variation can be reduced and the overall quality of health care can be improved.

Disease Management

The term "disease management" was first coined in the early 1990s by the Boston Consulting Group to describe an organized approach to managing populations of patients with a specific chronic illness. However, several of the older staff and group model HMOs, such as Kaiser Permanente, Harvard Community Health Plan, and Group Health Cooperative of Puget Sound, created and offered programs for patients with diseases such as asthma, diabetes, and heart disease long before the notion of disease management was formalized and more widely adopted by managed care organizations.

Today there are many formal definitions of disease. One of the most widely used is endorsed by the Disease Management Association of America: "Disease management is a system of coordinated health care interventions and communications for populations with conditions in which patient self-care efforts are significant. Disease management: supports the physician or practitioner/patient relationship and plan of care, emphasizes prevention of exacerbations and complications utilizing evidence-based practice guidelines and patient empowerment strategies, and evaluates clinical, humanistic, and economic outcomes on an ongoing basis with the goal of improving overall health."[42]

The basic components of disease management programs are:

- Tools to identify patients with a specific disease
- A risk stratification methodology to target patients with the highest risk of an exacerbation of their disease and/or a related hospitalization
- Clinical guidelines that are used by case managers to proactively support patients in self-managing their illness
- Patient education interventions
- Reports that inform physicians of any "gaps" in care or medical therapy
- A methodology to measure and report outcomes (clinical, utilization, financial, health status, and patient satisfaction)
- An information system that enable case managers to track clinical data on the patients they are following
- For some diseases, a remote patient monitoring capability (e.g., an electronic scale for patients with heart failure that reports daily weights to a case manager over the internet)

Health plans have most commonly implemented disease management programs for diabetes, asthma, heart failure, and coronary heart disease. Smaller numbers of plans have targeted high-risk pregnancy, depression, end-stage renal disease, HIV/AIDS, and COPD.[43] Recently, large self-insured employers have begun to implement similar programs for their employees in an attempt to reduce rapidly increasing medical costs and to increase employee productivity.

Managed care organizations and employers focus on these specific diseases for one of two reasons: there is an opportunity to save money by preventing costly hospitalizations (e.g., heart failure, diabetes, coronary heart disease) or there is an opportunity to dramatically improve outcomes and quality (e.g., asthma, high-risk maternity). These rationales are not mutually exclusive; many disease management programs are created with the goal of simultaneously improving quality and reducing medical costs.

Disease management programs can be challenging to implement. Most barriers to successful implementation fall into one of three categories: lack of strong physician leadership, failure to align incentives, or failure to address operational issues.[44] Despite these challenges, disease management programs are producing impressive improvements in quality and, for some diseases, are reducing costs. For example, multiple studies have documented significant reductions in hospital utilization (an important outcome measure) and decreased costs for patients with congestive heart failure.[45-47]

As leaders in health care, physicians need to understand that the need to improve quality is more important than ever, that our health care system does not deliver the optimal level of quality, and that we now have the methodologies and tools to significantly improve quality. We are entering an era in which employers, the government, and consumers are holding the profession accountable for medical errors and sub-optimal quality— not just for the cost of medical care. The development of integrated and comprehensive quality management programs using some of the tools described in this chapter—designed and run by clinicians—will be the best approach to improving the quality of medical care.

References

1. Committee on Quality of Health Care in America, Institute of Medicine. *To Err Is Human: Building a Safer Health System.* Washington, D.C.: National Academy Press, 1999. (www.nap.edu)

2. Committee on Quality of Health Care in America, Institute of Medicine. *Crossing the Quality Chasm: A New Health System for the 21st Century* Washington, D.C.: National Academy Press, 2002. (www.nap.edu)

3. Watson Wyatt Worldwide. "Creating a Sustainable Health Care Program: Eighth Annual Washington Business Group on Health/Watson Wyatt Survey Report, 2003. (www.watsonwyatt.com/research/resrender.asp?id=w-640&page=1)

4. www.wbgh.org

5. www.pbgh.org

6. www.leapfroggroup.org

7. Nash, D. *Connecting with the New Health Care Consumer.* Gaithersburg, Md.: Aspen Publishers, 2001.

8. Donabedian, A. *Defining and Measuring the Quality of Health Care.* Assessing Quality Health Care: Perspectives for Clinicians, Wenzel, R., Editor. Baltimore, Md.: Williams & Wilkins, 1992.

9. Nash, D., and Goldfield, N. "Information Needs of Purchasers." *In Providing Quality Care: The Challenge to Clinicians.* Nash, D., and Goldfield, N., Editors. Philadelphia, Pa.: American College of Physicians, 1989.

10. U.S. Congress, Office of Technology Assessment. *The Quality of Medical Care: Information for Consumers.* Washington, D.C.: U.S. Government Printing Office, June 1988, OTA-H-386

11. Nash, D. *Buying Value in Health Care.* Washington, D.C.: National Association of Manufacturers, 1992

12. Chassin, M., and others. "The Urgent Need to Improve Health Care Quality." *JAMA* 280(11):1000-5, Sept. 16, 1998.

13. Wennberg, J., and others. "Hospital Use and Mortality Among Medicare Beneficiaries in Boston and New Haven." *New England Journal of Medicine* 321(17):1168-73, Oct. 26, 1989.

14. Wennberg, J. "The Paradox of Appropriate Care." *JAMA* 258(18):2568-9, Nov. 13, 1987.

15. Wennberg, J. "Dealing with Medical Practice Variations: A Proposal for Action." *Health Affairs* 3(2):6-32, Summer 1984.

16. Brook, R., and others. *Appropriateness of Acute Medical Care for the Elderly: An Analysis of the Literature.* Santa Monica, Calif.: RAND Corporation, 1989.

17. Merrick, N., and others. "Use of Carotid Endarterectomy in Five California Veterans Administration Medical Centers." *JAMA* 256(18):2531-5, Nov. 14, 1986.

18. Chassin, M., and others. "Does Inappropriate Use Explain Geographic Variations in the Use of Health Care Services?" *JAMA* 258(18):2533-7, Nov. 13, 1987.

19. Doughty, R., and others. "Effects of Beta-Blocker Therapy on Mortality in Patients with Heart Failure. A Systematic Overview of Randomized Controlled Trials." *European Heart Journal* 18(4):560-5, April 1997.

20. Krum, H., and others. "Effects of Initiating Carvedilol in Patients with Severe Chronic Heart Failure: Results from the COPERNICUS Study." *JAMA* 289(6):712-8, Feb. 12, 2003.

21. Moseley, J., and others. "A Controlled Trial of Arthroscopic Surgery for Osteoarthritis of the Knee." *New England Journal of Medicine* 347(2):81-88, July 11, 2002.

22. Donabedian, A. "The Quality of Care: How Can It Be Assessed?" *JAMA* 260(12):1743-8, Sept. 23-30, 1988.

23. Laffel, G., and Blumenthal, D. "The Case for Using Industrial Quality Management Science in Health Care Organizations." *JAMA* 262(20):2869-73, Nov. 24, 1989.

24. Juran, J. *Juran's Quality Handbook,* McGraw-Hill Professional; 5th edition, New York, N.Y.: McGraw-Hill, 1998.

25. Deming, W. *Out of the Crisis.* Cambridge, Mass.: MIT Press, 2000.

26. Berwick, D., and others. *Curing Health Care: New Strategies for Quality Improvement.* San Francisco, Calif.: Jossey-Bass Publishers, 1990.

27. "The Role of Hospital Leadership in the Continuous Improvement of Patient Care Quality." *Journal for Healthcare Quality* 14(5):8-14,22, Sept.-Oct. 1992

28. Jencks, S., and Wilensky, G. "The Health Care Quality Improvement Initiative: A New Approach to Quality Assurance in Medicine." *JAMA* 268(7):900-3, Aug. 19, 1992.

29. www.ihi.org

30. www.ihi.org/idealized/idcop/

31. Berwick, D. "Continuous Improvement as an Ideal in Health Care." *New England Journal of Medicine* 320(1):53-6, Jan. 5, 1989.

32. Plsek, P. "A Primer on Quality Improvement Tools." In *Curing Health Care: New Strategies for Quality Improvement,* Berwick, D., and others, Editors. San Francisco, Calif.: Jossey-Bass Publishers, 1990.

33. O'Rourke, L.. "Benchmarking: A New Tool for Quality Improvement in Healthcare." *Quality Letter for Healthcare Leaders* 4(7):1-9, Sept. 1992

34. Ziegenfuss, J. "Organizational Barriers to Quality Improvement in Medical and Healthcare Organizations." *American Journal of Medical Quality* 6(4):115-22, Winter 1991.

35. Coffey, R., and others. "An Introduction to Critical Paths." *Quality Management in Health Care* 1(1):45-54, Fall 1992

36. Cabana, M., and others. "Why Don't Physicians Follow Clinical Practice Guidelines?: A Framework for Improvement." *JAMA* 282(15):1458-65, Oct. 20, 1999.

37. www.chsd.org

38. www.guideline.gov.

39. Ellwood, P. "Outcomes Management: A Technology of Patient Experiences." *New England Journal of Medicine* 318(23):1549-56, June 9, 1988.

40. Winslow, R. "Report Card on Quality and Efficiency of HMOs May Provide a Model for Others." *Wall Street Journal,* March 9, 1993, page B1.

41. Reinhardt, U. "The Importance of Quality in the Debate on National Health Policy." In *Health Care Quality Management for the 21st Century,* Couch, J., Editor. Tampa, Fla.: American College of Physician Executives, 1991.

42. www.dmaa.org

43. Welch, W., and others. "Disease Management Practices of Health Plans." *American Journal of Managed Care,* 8(4):353-61, April 2002.

44. Leider, H., and Krizan, K. "Disease Management—A Great Idea, but Can You Implement It? *Disease Management* 4(3):111-9, Fall 2001.

45. Clarke, J., and Nash, D. "The Effectiveness of Heart Failure Disease Management: Initial Findings from a Comprehensive Program." *Disease Management* 5(4):215-23, Winter 2002.

46. Krumholtz, H., and others. "Randomized Controlled Trial of an Education and Support Intervention to Prevent Readmission of Patients with Heart Failure. *Journal of American College of Cardiology* 39(1):83-9, Jan. 2, 2002.

47. Vaccaro, J., and others. "Utilization Reduction, Cost Savings, and Return on Investment for the PacifiCare Chronic Heart Failure Program." *Disease Management* 4(3):131-42, Fall 2001.

Harry L. Leider, MD, MBA, FACPE is the Chief Medical Officer and Senior Vice President of Ameritox, a national pain medication monitoring company. Prior to joining Ameritox he was Chief Medical Officer of XLHealth, a national disease management firm and Medicare health plan. He is a core faculty member of the American College of Physician Executives.

David B. Nash, MD, MBA, FACPE is Dr. Raymond C. and Doris N. Grandon Professor of Health Policy and Medicine at Jefferson Medical College of Thomas Jefferson University in Philadelphia. His is also Director of the Office of Health Policy and Clinical Outcomes, Thomas Jefferson University Hospital, and Dean for Health Policy, Jefferson Medical College, both in Philadelphia, Pa.

Chapter 7

To Err Is Human:
The Institute of Medicine Report Revisited — How Are We Doing?

by Frederic G. Jones, MD, FACPE

American Medicine enters the second decade after the 1999 IOM Report *To Err Is Human*.[1] the first of its 11-volume "Quality Chasm" series on improving patient care and avoiding mistakes that cited research estimating as many as 98,000 Americans die annually from preventable medical errors. *To Err is Human* attracted a flurry of media attention and political scrutiny—as well as criticism from physicians who said the estimate was too high. It also helped catalyze the modern patient safety movement, but to what end?

Are we really better today at preventing mistakes and safeguarding our systems from causing harm than we were 10 years ago? In the earlier edition of this book, the author reported on the state of patient safety on the fifth anniversary of this report. In ensuing years it was found that hospitals have made less than hoped for progress in improving patient safety. Hospital patient safety systems are not yet meeting IOM recommendations. While most hospitals had made substantial progress in surgical areas, that was not the case for medication safety, despite a long history of error prevention efforts. Far fewer than expected of responding hospitals reported having a fully implemented computerized physician order entry (CPOE) system. While hospitals showed improvements in specific areas, there were setbacks in every area surveyed. It was recommended that hospitals conduct their own surveys to assess progress in each of the major areas. In addition, more aggressive efforts are needed outside hospital systems—for example, heightened consumer awareness of quality and safety through performance reporting and mandatory public reporting of hospital errors.

This state existed despite the recommendations of such physician organizations as the American College of Physicians. ACP believes that the public has a right to expect health care that is safe and effective. The profession is responsible to individual patients and to the public to continuously seek to improve the quality of medical care and make sure that health care services are provided as safely as possible. The College believes that the focus must be on reform of the system, not punishment of individuals.

A colleague, Schimmel, had written of the hazards of hospitalization in a now classic report. This was a prospective assessment of risk involving all members of the internal medicine house staff at Yale in 1960-61 during his year as chief resident. This report provoked a great deal of thought but few demonstrated changes. In addition, there was little media attention.[2]

A report, *Patient Safety at Ten: Unmistakable Progress, Troubling Gaps* issued on December 1, 2009, in the policy journal *Health Affairs*, said patient safety efforts since 1999 deserve a B-minus grade, compared with a C-plus for 2004.[3] The report cited improvements in error reporting and quality initiatives led by the Institute for Healthcare Improvement, the Agency for Healthcare Research and Quality, the Joint Commission, and others. But, the report said, safety gains from health information technology have largely failed to materialize due to slow take-up, unintended consequences, and implementation problems.

The famed 2001 Institute of Medicine report, *Crossing the Quality Chasm*,[4,5] demonstrated that U.S. health care suffered from so many shortcomings that it scarcely warranted the name. These reports established a clear consensus: To arrive at health care that was high quality—that is, safe, effective, patient-centered, efficient, delivered on a timely basis, and devoid of disparities based on race or ethnicity—would require a Herculean effort to move the field across the abyss. As recently as April, 2011, it was fair to ask the question "Still Crossing The Quality Chasm—Or Suspended Over It? by Susan Dentzer, editor-in-chief of a thematic issue of *Health Affairs*.[6]

Unfortunately, according to recent data, it remains unclear whether, in the aggregate, efforts to reduce errors have translated into significant improvements in the overall safety of patients. The most specific problem areas continue to be complications from surgical procedures and drugs, as well as hospital-acquired infections. These are still the most common and most hazardous threats to patients in U.S. hospitals.

As a result of some enthusiastic efforts, hospital accreditation procedures and standards have become more rigorous, resident physician duty hours have been trimmed, hand-sanitizing gel dispensers in hospitals have multiplied and physician reimbursement has been linked increasingly with quality goals.

An AHRQ-funded report, *Designing Consumer Reporting Systems for Patient Safety*,[7] was developed for the purpose of making recommendations for an ideal reporting system that consumers would use to report experiences with patient safety events. The technical expert panel made recommendations based on a set of six research questions developed by AHRQ. One of the panel recommendations is that reporting systems should collect information on all types of events, ranging from near-miss and no-harm events to adverse events. The expert panel also recommends that information collected from consumers should include where a patient safety event occurred, what contributed to the event; whether or to whom an event was reported, what happened when an event was reported, and the impacts or consequences of the event.

A new series of reports by the Agency, *Closing the Quality Cap, Revisiting the State of the Science* (hereafter, the CQC Series),[8] continues to focus on improving the quality of health care through critical assessment of relevant evidence for selected settings, interventions, and clinical conditions. This series expands the topic terrain and marshals the knowledge of eight evidence-based practice centers (EPCs). These centers will review the literature for evidence and provide reports to target multiple audiences and associated uses, stating the science of quality and safety improvement.

However, there is some good news. Many states now require reporting of adverse events and some require public reporting of hospital-acquired infections, patient falls, or pressure ulcers. Medical residents' hours are now restricted to prevent errors caused by fatigue. Providers in many hospitals that normally compete have joined hands to standardize quality and safety metrics.

The Institute for Healthcare Improvement launched a number of safety strategies, including its "100,000 Lives Campaign." Following that campaign, the IHI launched its "5 Million Lives Campaign" to understand and address those medical mistakes, an estimated 40,000 per day, that injure patients and take a toll on their quality of life.

Another initiative of the IHI was "Getting the Board on Board."[9] These efforts to ensure greater involvement of the governing bodies in quality and patient safety have changed the agendas of many hospital and system boards. The author just completed a 5-year term as a board member of a not-for-profit critical access hospital in the mountains of western North Carolina. The board was concerned with evidence that this category of hospital was not performing as well as larger and urban hospitals. The board chose to create a board quality council to review patient safety and quality data. This included a dashboard for easy assessment by the board members, who were mainly lay persons. This success can be measured by the decision to place the quality council report as the first agenda item of each monthly board meeting. 2011 reports on hospital performance from the NC Center for Hospital Quality and Patient Safety Quality Dashboard for this hospital show all conditions in the top quartile!

There are some elements that are crucial for health care leaders following health care reform—the need to stay focused and vigilant about high quality and safe patient care. Recent surveys show that more health care organizations are putting patient safety among their top priorities. Original research and analysis in the *HealthLeaders Media Intelligence Report* [10] offers key insight from top health care executives and clinical leaders who are planning to devote more financial resources to patient safety programs. They say lack of communication skills poses the greatest risk to patient safety during handoffs and transitions of care when important patient care information is often lost. They agree that improved infection control practices are among the most important new initiatives designed to improve patient safety.

Providers are setting goals for their communities. Hospitals are starting to use the IHI "global trigger tool" to more accurately measure areas of care that might be causing avoidable harm, including the 28 adverse events now required to be reported.

Facilities were urged to adopt a "no-blame" system to encourage providers to report their own missteps, in the chance that the practice or situation might be easily repeated by a colleague. Disclosure of those mistakes and transparency have become acceptable at many facilities as well.

Central Line Associated Bloodstream Infections have been reduced.

Many facilities are using "checklists" before beginning surgery or a complex procedure.

The Centers for Medicare and Medicaid Services will no longer reimburse health facilities for the cost of caring for a patient with a preventable hospital-acquired infection.

More attention is being paid to physicians' diagnostic errors, and the importance of being candid with patients and patients' families when preventable errors occur.

Many significant challenges remain, but that may be changing. As described in a *New York Times* column, in the summer of 2011, nearly 1,000 surgeons, nurses and hospital administrators from across the country convened in Boston to discuss what is quickly becoming one of the most far-reaching of such efforts, the National Surgical Quality Improvement

Program (NSQIP) from the American College of Surgeons, the largest professional organization of surgeons.[11,12] With the average American undergoing nine operations in his or her lifetime, the implications of a program that can improve how patients do after surgery are enormous. The program is now used by surgeons at more than 400 institutions. Unlike most other quality programs, which gather data from insurance claims and coding data, it relies on information from patients' hospital charts and follows patients for 30 days. A detailed analysis, along with statistics comparing results with those of all other participating hospitals, is then sent back to participating hospitals. The efforts pay off. Within two years of adopting the program, almost 70 percent of hospitals decreased their mortality rates, and more than 80 percent decreased their complication rates.

The American College of Surgeons hopes eventually to collaborate with regulatory and federal agencies so that more hospitals, and patients, might be able to benefit. And it's working with participating hospitals to further refine the program. The College of Surgeons hopes to enlist at least 1,000 hospitals in the program. As part of the initiative, the ACS has released a series of videos that can be found on the ACS website, www.facs.org/quality.

Adherence to surgical care improvement measured by a composite infection prevention score, but not by individual measures, was linked to a lower probability of postoperative infection, according to the results of a retrospective cohort study reported in the June 23/30, 2010, issue of the *Journal of the American Medical Association*.[13] The Surgical Care Improvement Project (SCIP) aims to reduce surgical infectious complication rates through measurement and reporting of 6 infection-prevention process-of-care measures. However, an association between SCIP performance and clinical outcomes has not been demonstrated. None of the individual SCIP measures were significantly associated with a lower risk for infection.[14-19].

Certain types of medical errors are 46 percent less likely to occur at top-rated U.S. hospitals than at bottom-ranked hospitals, according to a new study. Health Grades researchers analyzed 40 million Medicare patient records from 2007 to 2009 and focused on 13 patient safety indicators, such as bed sores, bloodstream infections from catheters, foreign objects left in the body after procedures and excessive bleeding or bruising after surgery.

The patient safety indicators published by the U.S. Agency for Healthcare Research and Quality were used to identify preventable medical errors and the hospitals that were in the top 5 percent for avoiding those errors. Nationwide, hospitals varied widely in their performance, according to the annual Health Grades *Patient Safety in American Hospitals* report. Some hospitals have made significant improvements, but the fact remains that there are huge, life-and-death consequences associated with where a patient chooses to seek hospital care.The13 patient safety indicators included in the study were associated with $7.3 billion in additional costs, or $181 per Medicare patient hospitalization.

A decade ago, rates of hand hygiene in most American hospitals were shameful, often below 20%. As attention began to focus on unacceptably high rates of health care-associated infections, most organizations treated low hand-hygiene rates as a systems problem. Many launched "hand hygiene campaigns," accompanied by internal dissemination of hand-hygiene rates and admonitions by senior administrators to improve the rates (sometimes accompanied by financial incentives). Hand-gel dispensers were placed in or near every patient's room. A few institutions even brought in human-factors engineers to assess the overall hand-hygiene system and recommend process changes. To the degree that the failure to clean hands was due to flawed systems or provider ignorance, these actions made sense.

Despite these efforts, most hospitals continue to have hand-hygiene rates that range from 30 to 70%, and few have sustained rates over 80. It seems that in most U.S. hospitals, this answer is no longer the correct one. In 2011, low hand-hygiene rates are generally not a systems problem anymore; they are largely an accountability problem.[20]

In late 2008 the Joint Commission created its Center for Transforming Healthcare to work together with hospitals and systems that have mastered robust process improvement methods to apply these tools to vital safety and quality problems. Hand hygiene was the first problem addressed by a group of eight hospitals that worked with the center. Teams from the Joint Commission and the eight hospitals first agreed on how to measure hand hygiene, developed the measurement system, and proved its reliability. Applying the measurement system produced the first discovery: Baseline hand hygiene performance at the hospitals in April 2009 was a disappointingly low 48 percent.

Each hospital had a different set of important causes. The implications of this finding are important. A time-honored method of improving health care is the replication of "best practices." Using this approach, the eight hospitals reported in August 2010 that their aggregate performance for hand hygiene had risen to 81 percent—a rate they had sustained for 10 months.

Central line-related infections are an appropriate target for all clinical care systems, with dramatic reductions possible. AHRQ released a second report that highlights the progress that has been achieved by hospitals taking part in a national effort to reduce the incidence of central line-associated bloodstream infections (CLABSI) by implementing a Comprehensive Unit-based Safety Program (CUSP).

American hospital intensive care units cut central line-associated bloodstream infections by about 60% over nearly a decade, saving an estimated 27,000 lives and avoiding up to $1.8 billion in medical costs, said a new report from the Centers for Disease Control and Prevention.

"This is the first national success we have for patient safety in this country," said Peter J. Pronovost, MD, PhD. He is principal investigator of a bundle of central-line infection prevention techniques that in 2006 demonstrated success statewide in Michigan and has spread to nearly 1,000 hospitals in 43 states.

The CDC report, published in the March 4, 2011, *Morbidity and Mortality Weekly Report*, compared ICU bloodstream infection rates among the 260 hospitals reporting in 2001 with about 1,600 hospitals participating in the agency's National Healthcare Safety Network in 2009. Researchers used infection surveillance information and billing data on the number of days patients were on central lines to estimate the number of lives and dollars saved. About 25% of all patients with bloodstream infections die, the CDC said.

In 2002, the CDC issued guidelines on preventing bloodstream infections related to central lines. In Dr. Pronovost's work in Michigan, reported in the Dec. 28, 2006, issue of *The New England Journal of Medicine*, ICUs virtually eliminated these bloodstream infections by implementing better hand hygiene, using full-barrier precautions when inserting central venous catheters, cleaning the skin with chlorhexidine, avoiding the femoral site for catheter insertion and removing unnecessary catheters.

What has set apart the national effort to cut bloodstream infections is the scientific rigor with which it has been pursued, said Robert M. Wachter, MD, chief of the Division of Hospital Medicine at the University of California, San Francisco Medical Center.

"No one woke up one day and said, 'Here's the bundle,'" Dr. Wachter said. "We had to study each element of the bundle and demonstrate that using barrier precautions or certain line-insertion techniques really worked. It took many years to demonstrate that."

The AHA is responsible for administering a $5.8 million Agency for Healthcare Research & Quality grant to implement Dr. Pronovost's Comprehensive Unit-Based Safety Program, known as On the CUSP.

Central-line infections are a problem not only in the ICU. They also are common in other areas of the hospital and among patients on dialysis. The CDC report estimated there were 23,000 central-line infections among inpatients outside the ICU in 2009 and 37,000 bloodstream infections among hemodialysis outpatients in 2008. The CDC did not have comparative data for earlier in the decade.

Among dialysis patients, the challenge has been to encourage more of them to steer clear of catheters, as It is difficult to prevent infections among patients using a catheter for dialysis three times a week. Since 2003, the Fistula First Breakthrough Coalition has sought to increase the number of patients opting for an arteriovenous fistula.

A Feb. 8 coalition report showed AV fistula use among dialysis patients rose from 34.1% in 2003 to 57.4% in 2010, but more than 81% of patients start dialysis using a catheter—raising the risk of bloodstream infections.

Experts said the lessons learned from the national success with central-line infections could help slash catheter-related urinary tract infections, ventilator-associated pneumonia and surgical-site infections. One element critical to bringing the science to the bedside is putting doctors and other health professionals in charge of implementation, said Dr. Pronovost, director of the Division of Adult Critical Care Medicine at The Johns Hopkins Hospital in Baltimore.

A new study by UNC researchers finds that an inexpensive set of infection control measures could potentially save many thousands of lives and billions of dollars. At any given time, one of every 20 hospital patients has a hospital-acquired infection, according to the U.S. Department of Health and Human Services. This leads to an estimated 99,000 deaths in the U.S. each year and up to $33 billion in preventable health care costs. The new study by University of North Carolina at Chapel Hill researchers finds that adopting an inexpensive set of infection control measures could potentially save many thousands of lives and billions of dollars. The study appears in the September 2011 issue of *Health Affairs*. Strict enforcement of standard hand hygiene practices was one of three interventions tested in the study.

"These two initiatives, targeting ventilator-associated pneumonias and central line-associated bloodstream infections, involved simple steps that lead to dramatic reductions in not only the targeted infections, but also mortality and costs," said Bradford D. Harris, MD, who led the study while serving as an associate professor of anesthesiology and pediatrics in the UNC School of Medicine. He is now a medical officer at the U.S. Food and Drug Administration in Washington. The study was conducted in the Pediatric Intensive Care Unit at North Carolina Children's Hospital, which is one of the five University of North Carolina Hospitals. The study tested three interventions aimed at preventing and reducing hospital acquired infections.

The first intervention was strict enforcement of standard hand hygiene practices on the unit. All health care workers are expected to wash their hands with soap and running water or an alcohol-based rub on entering and leaving a patient's room, before putting on and after removing gloves, and before and after any task that involves touching potentially contaminated surfaces or body fluids. The second intervention was implementing a bundle of measures aimed at preventing ventilator-associated pneumonia. Examples included elevating the head of the patient's bed while the patient is receiving breathing assistance from a ventilator, giving the patient daily breaks from sedation and then—while the patient was unsedated—assessing whether or not the patient is ready to come off the ventilator, and providing daily oral care (teeth brushing, mouth washes, etc.) with a long-lasting antiseptic.

The final intervention was ensuring compliance with guidelines for the use and maintenance of central-line catheters. Examples included using sponges impregnated with an antiseptic, using catheters impregnated with antibiotics whenever possible, and performing two assessments per day of whether patients with central-line catheters still needed them.

Results of the study showed that patients admitted after these interventions were fully implemented got out of the hospital an average of two days earlier, their hospital stay cost about $12,000 less, and the number of patient deaths was reduced by two percentage points.

The costs for implementing these measures were modest. Examples include roughly $21 a day for oral care kits and about 60 cents a day for antiseptic patches and hand sanitizers. But adoption of the three interventions collectively could save this single hospital unit an estimated $12 million a year, the study found. If replicated nationwide, these measures potentially could save thousands of lives and billions of dollars each year. The study concluded that measures such as these have the potential to save both lives and money and will improve the care of all patients.

A similar argument can be made about other commonsense safety practices, such as using a checklist to reduce bloodstream infections, marking the surgical site to prevent wrong-site surgery, and performing a preoperative "time-out." One continues to hear many examples of physicians who fail (and sometimes even refuse) to perform such procedures. The costs of the failure to enforce safety standards are real. For example, approximately 4000 wrong-side surgeries are performed annually in the United States. Although it is likely that most such errors are preventable with adherence to the Universal Protocol (which includes surgical-site marking and a pre-operative time-out), physicians frequently skip some required steps. Many experts believe that many, if not most, of the estimated 100,000 annual deaths from health care-associated infections in the United States could be prevented by strict adherence to infection-control practices, including hand hygiene.

Today, some health care organizations are adopting the new generation of industrial quality methods and applying them to issues of clinical safety and quality. The new approaches—Six Sigma, lean management, and change management—are far more robust in their ability to solve difficult safety and quality problems. We refer to them, collectively, as "robust process improvement." Taken together, they are a systematic approach to dissecting complex safety problems and guiding organizations to deploy highly effective solutions. The power of these tools lies in their systematic approach, which involves the following: reliably measuring the magnitude of a problem; identifying the root causes of the problem and measuring the importance of each cause; finding solutions for the most important causes; proving the effectiveness of those solutions; and deploying programs to ensure sustained improvements over time. Robust process improvement enables health care organizations to avoid crucial failures common in many efforts to improve clinical quality.

The Joint Commission has produced tools to spread the knowledge gained from improvement projects to all of the health care organizations it has accredited. In the fall of 2011, all accredited organizations will have access to the wrong site solutions through the Targeted Solutions Tool (TST).

AnMed Health joined seven other hospitals and ambulatory surgical centers in volunteering for this project. Since 10,000 surgeries were performed in this regional medical center each year, the project team felt a unique opportunity to develop useful tools to assess and improve patient safety. Several opportunities for improvement were identified, such as phone- and paper-based scheduling processes. Capturing the demographic information made the scheduling more accurate. As is often the case, ineffective communication and distractions in the operating room contributed to increasing the risk of wrong site surgery. In addition, a time out without full participation by all key people in the operating room was identified as another contributing factor that increased risk. A new program was initiated to name each month the surgeons who embrace the opportunity and call time outs enthusiastically on their own.

It's critical to show staff the positive effects of near-miss reporting. It's also a good idea to publicly and consistently reward those who "see/experience something and say something." A good example is one surgical suite in Johns Hopkins Hospital in Baltimore that implemented its Good Catch Awards. After 24 months, the health center provided a table of 27 good catches that shows how systems were changed in response to the catch, including one that led to a national recall of an improperly labeled drug that lead to look-alike medication errors. Clinicians honored with an award receive public recognition with wall boards on the surgical suite. The system is not yet implemented hospital-wide, but continues at the Weinberg OR Suite at Johns Hopkins Hospital.

Another focus of intense interest is optimal medication management. These processes range from medication reconciliation to the utilization of advanced technology such as CPOE and bar-coding. Particularly important is the prevention of errors at time of transitions, such as transfers between units and discharge from the hospital.[21-25]

By now, most of us involved in patient safety understand the importance of reporting, collecting, and analyzing near misses. Before the failure to adhere to safety standard results in individual blame and punishment, we must not forget that such failures often are due to systems factors. Dysfunctional systems, which are sometimes created by providers or administrators who lack essential training in human factors and systems engineering, may make it too hard to adhere to the practice, inviting workarounds. Systems thinking remain a powerful concept, and expecting strict adherence to safety standards before addressing the relevant systems issues would be a mistake.

As we enter the second decade of the safety movement, while the science regarding improving systems must continue to mature, the urgency of the task also demands that we stop averting our eyes from the need to balance "no blame" and accountability. Finding this balance will be challenging. Having our own profession deem some behaviors as unacceptable, with clear consequences, will serve as a vivid example of our professionalism, and thus represent our best protection against such outside intrusions. But the main reason to find the right balance between "no blame" and individual accountability is that doing so will save lives.

Traditional efforts to detect adverse events have focused on voluntary reporting and tracking of errors. However, public health researchers have established that only 10 to 20 percent of errors are ever reported and, of those, 90 to 95 percent cause no harm to patients. Hospitals need a more effective way to identify events that do cause harm to patients in order to quantify the degree and severity of harm, and to select and test changes to reduce harm.

The IHI Global Trigger Tool for Measuring Adverse Events provides an easy-to-use method for accurately identifying adverse events (harm) and measuring the rate of adverse events over time. Tracking adverse events over time is a useful way to tell if changes being made are improving the safety of the care processes. The Trigger Tool methodology includes a retrospective review of a random sample of patient records using "triggers" (or clues) to identify possible adverse events. Many hospitals have used this tool to identify adverse events, to measure the level of harm from each adverse event, and to identify areas for improvement in their organizations.

How far we have come since then—and how far we still have to go—are the subjects of a thematic issue of *Health Affairs*, sponsored by the Robert Wood Johnson Foundation (which has itself made huge investments over the past decade in its Aligning Forces for Quality initiative). As a number of articles in the issue demonstrate, there's no doubt we've made progress—but it's also clear that making any headway has been agonizingly slow. If ever the state of high-quality health care appeared to be an achievable end point, we recognize now that—to paraphrase Ralph Waldo Emerson—quality, like life, is not a destination but a journey.

Closing the Quality Gap: Revisiting the State of the Science -- Series Overview Patient Safety Monitor, March 1, 2011, eliminating preventable harm by defining it. Defining what is "preventable" proved to be much more difficult; many saw it as a subjective term. The injury results from failure to provide care to the existing institutional standard OR reasonable adaptations to the existing standard can be introduced that would be expected to decrease the risk of future injury by the same mechanism. This would mean that, for example, a failure to complete any piece of the hospital's ventilator-associated pneumonia bundle on any particular occasion would mean that harm was preventable. The next hurdle was understanding how to track preventable harm throughout the system. Preventing medical errors and patient harm is a top priority for most hospitals. Physicians, nurses, and other clinicians do not enter their professions to produce poor outcomes. However, medicine is an inherently risky business, and sometimes patients are harmed. Informing patients and their families of harm—which may or may not have resulted from an error—is always difficult. We need to know whether the process is under control and can repeatedly produce outcomes that meet our specifications. In addition, we need to know whether the process has caused harm in the past and whether there are areas that could potentially cause harm in the future.

Moreover, the available evidence suggests that the risk of harmful error in health care may be increasing. In a JAMA commentary, "Exploring the Harmful Effects of Health Care,"[26-27] we are reminded that harm may occur as a direct or indirect consequence of health care. Direct harm includes adverse physical and emotional effects, generally to individuals, as a by-product of health care delivery. Indirect harm is a collateral effect on individuals and communities not directly involved in care, Excess health care costs may induce harm by competing with other health-producing services. This is described in a current review article in PEJ entitled *Over treatment in Health Care: How Much is Too Much?*[28] It is a fact that cost of health care in the United States far exceeds that of other industrialized nations, due, in part, to overutilization of health resources. Unnecessary care can cause both physical and emotional harm, both having effects on patient well-being. This may require a culture change of clinical care clinicians, health system leaders, payers, purchasers, and, above all, patients, to be effective and capable of producing clinical outcomes that are of value.

As new devices, equipment, procedures, and drugs are added to our therapeutic arsenal, the complexity of delivering effective care increases. Complexity greatly increases the likelihood of error, especially in systems that perform at low levels of reliability.

The most complex health care is delivered in hospitals, which are populated by patients whose severity and acuity of illness have been increasing inexorably. This is because many of the least sick patients no longer require hospital stays to receive the care they need. For example, patients are no longer admitted to hospitals for diagnostic evaluations. Surgical procedures previously performed only in hospitals with considerable lengths of stay are now routinely and safely done in ambulatory settings. Treatments such as long-term intravenous infusions for combating certain serious infections are performed safely at home. Thus, we face the intersection of two interrelated trends: Hospitals house patients who are increasingly vulnerable to harm due to error and the complexity of the care hospitals now provide increases the likelihood of those errors.

An editorial in *JAMA* and FDA warnings have identified numbers of patients undergoing radiation for diagnosis and treatment to have received excess doses of radiation.[29] More than 250 patients treated received up to 8 times the expected dose of radiation during computer-assisted tomography perfusion scans. The Agency and the Joint Commission are defining new safety goals to prevent these outcomes. It is not yet clear whether human error or design flaws in machines contributed to these adverse events.

In early October, the FDA warned health care workers that it had received reports of 206 patients receiving excess doses of radiation from computed tomographic (CT) scans used to diagnose stroke over an 18-month period at Cedars-Sinai Medical Center in Los Angeles. Since then the agency and local health officials have identified at least 50 more affected patients. Additional cases were identified at Cedars-Sinai and two other California hospitals, as well as at least one hospital in Alabama.

Some of the overexposed patients developed skin redness or experienced hair loss, and all of the exposed patients may be at increased risk of developing certain cancers or cataracts in the months or years following their scans, said Charles Finder, MD, associate director of the division of mammography quality and radiation programs at the FDA's CDRH.

To help prevent such outcomes, the agency is urging facilities and CT technicians to redouble their efforts to ensure that proper radiation doses are used. The agency recommends that facilities determine whether any of their patients have received inappropriate doses, review their dosing protocols, and implement quality-control measures to verify that dosing protocols are being followed for each scan.

In the therapeutic radiation area, the Radiation Oncology Organization and the FDA have committed to a patient protection plan that will improve safety and quality and reduce the chances of medical errors. A central database will be created for the reporting of errors involving linear accelerators and CT scanners used in the treatment plans for cancer patients. In addition, the development of clinical registries, such as the National Cardiovascular Registry, have the capability of identifying error potential, as well as the appropriate selection of patients undergoing procedures. In a recent study in JAMA, it was determined that the majority of patients are appropriately selected for percutaneous coronary intervention (PCI). This is especially true of PCIs performed in the acute setting (98.6 percent). However, for non-acute indications, 11.6 percent were categorized as inappropriate, with substantial variation noted across hospitals.

Another editorial was entitled "Achieving Meaningful Device Surveillance from Action to Proaction."[30] A number of devices have been removed from the market. However, the studies raised questions as to the adequacy of the U.S. device approval and post-approval device surveillance safety net. The VA system provides an example of national, proactive point-of-care surveillance by its Clinical Assessment, Reporting and Tracking (CART) system. As the U.S. moves to achieve "meaningful use' of electronic health records, we may be better equipped to detect these risks.

Technology at the bedside may aid the future of patient safety and quality. Many hospitals have implemented electronic medical records (EMR) or are currently doing so, and the federal government provides incentives for using this technology in a meaningful way. However, some new technology suggests the potential to go even further. Individual clinicians already know this; they use tablets and smart phones to communicate and take advantage of useful, informative applications in a more portable way during their shifts.

The goal of choosing, developing, and implementing healthcare technology is to make the right thing to do the easy thing to do. There's a false sense in some hospitals that spending money on technology equates to safety. In reality, that's not always the case.

The idea is to ensure that technology at the bedside is implemented with human factors in mind, meaning it should make things easier for frontline caregivers, be easy to use, and not become an obstacle to efficient and safe work. One of the biggest impacts you can have on quality and patient safety is human factors, Work should be designed to make it very hard to fail. In addition, the next major frontier may involve physicians and other practitioners more directly with an increasing emphasis on diagnostic errors.[31]

The need for major improvements in safety and quality has never been greater. Yet current approaches are not producing the pace, breadth, or magnitude of improvement that all stakeholders desire. Along with a number of other observers, we believe that it is essential to look outside health care for solutions. Specifically; we should first get a clear picture of how complex organizations establish and maintain extremely high levels of safety. Then we must apply the lessons we learn from them to health care.

The study of "high reliability"—or consistent performance at high levels of safety over long periods of time—began with investigations of organizations that manage extreme hazards with exemplary safety records, far better than those in health care today. Today we have studies of many different "high-reliability organizations," including the nuclear power industry, the commercial air travel system, and the flight decks of aircraft carriers. These studies have revealed several common key features that facilitate the maintenance of consistent excellence. These features incorporate a "collective mindfulness," which is a dominant attitude or cultural feature that all high-reliability organizations display.

What exactly is mindfulness? In *Teaching Mindfulness: A Practical Guide for Clinicians and Educators*, authors Donald McCown, Diane Reibel, and Marc Micozzi attempt to answer that question and to propose methods for teaching mindfulness, not only for health care professionals but also for patients. For this reason, the authors believe that clinicians should know as much as they can about mindfulness.

The authors favor Jon Kabat-Zinn's definition of mindfulness: "paying attention in a particular way: on purpose, in the present moment, nonjudgmentally" and point out that, "The three axioms of intention, attention, and attitude...are not sequential but rather engaged simultaneously in the process of mindfulness

Our failure to create real accountability for patient safety partly represents a fundamental misunderstanding regarding both how other, safer industries carry out their safety activities and the nature of errors. It is true that most errors are innocent slips committed by competent and committed caregivers and are best dealt with by focusing on improving systems rather than people. But as James Reason, the father of modern error theory and "systems thinking," emphasizes, every safe industry has transgressions that are firing offenses. The pilot who neglects to use a checklist before takeoff would not be allowed to fly (not to mention that the copilot would never agree to take off). Although finding the right balance between "no blame" and accountability is tricky for all caregivers, we believe it is particularly challenging in cases involving physicians.

Medical teams should take a lesson from airplane crews, a study in the *Archives of Surgery* concludes.[32] Medical personnel who used procedural checklists modeled after preflight checklists used by airplane crews were more likely to report safety-related incidents and feel empowered to address safety issues. The introduction of checklist-based programs, known in the aviation industry as "crew resource management programs," or CRMs, was accompanied by an increase in self-initiated reports of safety breaches among medical staff, from 709 per quarter in 2002 to 1,481 per quarter in 2008 among teams using the checklists. The introduction of CRM training, combined with other initiatives, enhances personal commitment to patient safety and appears to alter behaviors relative to checklist use and self-reporting. In addition to aviation principles, an interesting performance report from the U.S. Coast Guard describes high performance on a "square rigger."[33]

An IOM Roundtable, *On Value and Science-Driven Health Care Engineering: A Learning Health Care System* investigated how systems engineering has been successfully applied in three industries and sought to understand which lessons might be applied to the transformation of the sociologically and technologically complex health care sector. Implicit in the discussions was the importance of bold leadership in driving reform, the imperative of having clarity of mission, the merits of developing strong metrics and sharing results widely, and the value of investing in people.

John J. Nance, founding member of the National Patient Safety Foundation, reported on a rich set of systems reforms that has been achieved by the aviation industry. Nance summarized elements of aviation's use of engineering principles, including critical feedback systems associated with detecting and managing mechanical problems and the notion of "exquisite redundancy." The airlines built a system around the assumptions that humans are imperfect and that systems can be structured to correct—and even anticipate—human errors through training programs, procedure standardization, and variable minimization. He described the need for health care systems to plan for and expect failure in every aspect as well as the need for acceptance of these realities operationally and culturally. The wide scope and variety of engineering experiences adopted in aviation could be directly applicable to health care, legitimizing and inculcating known best practices, eliminating the need to reinvent every procedure, and providing operational buffers against human fallibility in order to allow for safer care delivery systems, Nance said.

The author with several other colleagues endeavored to interest hospitals and medical staffs in considering human factors engineering when designing patient safety projects. This stemmed from experiences as a flight surgeon and accident investigation team member. A collaborative effort with the director of CRM for a major airline elicited interest, but minimal implementation using the aviation industry model. Some years later, a surgical colleague at AnMed, who was an instrument-rated pilot and flight examiner, teamed up with a senior commercial pilot, again endeavoring to promote aviation-based team training to elicit sustainable behavioral change. Once more, only limited acceptance was found, suggesting major cultural objections by surgeons and other procedualists. Interestingly, the author had found a procedural checklist useful while performing cardiac catheterizations in the 1970s!

In 2007, a Harvard Medical School surgeon wrote an article in *The New Yorker* magazine that raised a lot of eyebrows. If surgery units would follow a very simple checklist, wrote Atul Gawande, MD, it would both save lives and lessen complications. Such a checklist was being promoted and used by Johns Hopkins critical care specialist Peter Pronovost, MD, he said, and it had made a remarkable difference. They are focused, brief, actionable, verbal, collaborative—and tested. They make a surgical team's life easier. More important, they have been proven to reduce surgical morbidity and mortality significantly. The checklists are a simple way to keep highly trained specialists focused on the complex procedures only they understand, without losing sight of the equally important fundamentals of taking care of patients during surgery.

According to the Centers for Disease Control and Prevention, there are somewhere upwards of 53 million outpatient and 46 million inpatient surgeries in the U.S. every year. Just think: If we can nudge the quality needle upward even a tiny bit, we can make a difference in many people's lives.

In their own way, the checklists actually underscore the complexity of what we do. Their success reflects the need to keep things as simple as possible where we can, in the midst of our very complicated world of science and technology. As Dr. Gawande points out in his book *The Checklist Manifesto*, something as simple as a checklist is a hard sell to a profession like ours. However, checklists are used routinely by pilots and in a variety of other industries. They are used because they work.

Michigan hospitals that implemented checklists to prevent central line-associated bloodstream infections in their intensive care units saw an average tenfold return on their investment in patient safety, said a study published in the September/October issue of the *American Journal of Medical Quality*. Each catheter-related bloodstream infection costs a Michigan hospital $36,500 to treat, on average, but implementing the checklist program costs only about $3,375 per infection avoided. More than 100 Michigan ICUs were able to cut bloodstream infections by an average of two-thirds, with many hospitals eliminating the infections entirely. On average, each hospital saved about $1.1 million a year by implementing the patient safety program, the study said. The patient safety "bundle" now being spread to hospitals nationwide costs each hospital an average of $161,000 to put into place, mostly for staff time.

Human factors engineering (HFE) is defined by the Human Factors and Ergonomics Society as the "scientific discipline concerned with the understanding of interactions among humans and other elements of a system, and the profession that applies theory, principles, data, and other methods to design in order to optimize human well-being and overall system performance." Although other high-reliability industries such as aviation and nuclear power have utilized HFE principles for decades, health care only recently began looking to HFE when designing processes and systems.

Creating a "culture of safety" is a concept that many health care facilities have become familiar with in the past five years. A culture of safety is one that deemphasizes individual blame and looks at errors from a systems perspective. James Reason, one of the most well-known thought leaders on the topic of human error, brought his idea of the "Swiss cheese model" to healthcare to explain how errors can occur in high-reliability organizations.[34-5] Reason talks about the "blunt end and the sharp end"—the blunt end is the organizational factors: staffing, turnover, poor policies, poor leadership, poor management, leading to the sharp-end problems, which are the nurse and the patient, or doctor and the patient. It's the person who interacts directly with the patient that is the recipient of all of those blunt-end problems.

Other human factors under scrutiny and change are cataloged in a *New York Times* piece, "*The Phantom Menace of Sleep Deprived Doctors.*" It now appears that the reduction in resident work hours has had less than expected improvement in patient safety studies. However, the emotional stress and physical exhaustion of house staff, especially in the first year of training, continues to be documented. In this national study of internal medicine residents, suboptimal QOL and symptoms of burnout were common. Symptoms of burnout were associated with higher debt and were less frequent among international medical graduates.

The April 2011 issue of *Health Affairs* features an article titled "The Ongoing Quality Improvement Journey: Next Stop, High Reliability,"[36] highlights high reliability, which can be defined as consistent excellence over long periods of time. In the article, the authors point out that other industries have achieved high reliability and it is time for health care to do the same. The article talks about the three critical changes that health care must make to become a high-reliability industry:

1. The responsibility of leadership to make high reliability the priority
2. The importance of creating a culture of safety within an organization
3. The use of proven quality methods—Lean Six Sigma and change management (known together as robust process improvement™) – to systematically improve processes and avoid common, crucial failures

Health care quality and safety today are best characterized as showing pockets of excellence on specific measures or in particular services at individual health care facilities. In addition, more organizations than ever before are actively engaged in a wide variety of improvement efforts.

These include the Medicare quality improvement organizations and a number of state-based and specialty initiatives, such as the Cardiac Surgery Reporting System, which stimulates improvement in the outcomes of cardiovascular procedures by collecting and disseminating clinically valid data on risk-adjusted mortality rates by hospital and physician. Private organizations such as the Institute for Healthcare Improvement, the Robert Wood Johnson Foundation, and the Commonwealth Fund have played vital roles in facilitating improvement activities on the part of health care providers and communities.

Regional collaboratives of multiple stakeholders have invigorated local improvement efforts, as have numerous initiatives directed by large integrated delivery systems and medical centers. Federal initiatives emanating from the health reform law, such as programs to create accountable care organizations, may further accelerate progress.

What has eluded us thus far, however, is maintaining consistently high levels of safety and quality over time and across all health care services and settings. The pockets of excellence mentioned above coexist with enormously variable performance across the delivery system. Along with some progress, we are experiencing an epidemic of serious and preventable adverse events. These include patients' undergoing surgical procedures intended for others, fires in operating rooms, and patients' committing suicide while in the care of hospitals.

A characteristic of high-reliability organizations has been described as "collective mindfulness." This term describes how everyone in such organizations, both individually and together, is acutely aware that even small failures in safety protocols or processes can lead to catastrophic adverse outcomes. As a matter of routine, workers in these organizations are always searching for the smallest indication that the environment or a key safety process has changed in some way that might lead to failure, if some action is not taken to solve the problem. Continuously uncovering these safety concerns permits an organization to identify safety or quality problems at a stage when they are easily fixed. As suggested in error terminology—"Prevent, Intercept, Mitigate!" In health care we are too often in the position of investigating severe adverse events after they have injured patients, which means that we have missed opportunities to pinpoint and correct quality problems before they cause harm.

In addition high-reliability organizations have two other features in common. First, after organizations identify potential deficiencies in safety processes, they eliminate these deficiencies through the use of powerful tools to improve their processes. These are the tools of robust process improvement, described below.

Second, the organizations rely on a particular organizational culture to ensure the performance of improved safety processes over long periods and to remain constantly aware of the possibility of failure. This may be called "safety culture"; it is also described below. Leadership must make a commitment to the goal of high reliability, the organizational culture that supports high reliability must be fully implemented, and the tools of robust process improvement must be adopted. It is believed that the organizational culture that is so essential to establishing and maintaining high reliability in health care is the "safety culture" described by James Reason.[36] He posits that this culture involves three mutually reinforcing imperatives: trust, report, and improve. High-reliability organizations receive regular reports on potentially unsafe conditions, poorly functioning safety procedures, or simple changes in the environment that might lead to failures of safety systems.

In the 1990s health care organizations experimented with the industrial quality improvement tools of the time—specifically, the approaches of continuous quality improvement and total quality management. Some hospitals and systems were able to achieve some improvements in quality with those approaches. However, most of the improvements were in non-clinical areas, and the tools were largely ineffective in solving clinical safety and quality problems. methodology with Deming-based principles of quality improvement.

What practical steps can health care organizations take to achieve high reliability? It is recommended that they begin with a self-assessment that examines their organizational readiness in terms of the three components described above: leadership, safety culture, and the capacity to execute robust process improvement. Individual health care organizations that wish to make progress toward high reliability have chosen many different paths.

Many organizations outside of health care have been able to establish high levels of excellence in managing hazardous processes and to maintain those levels over long periods with rates of adverse events many times lower than occur commonly in health care. Can health care reach this state of high reliability and stay there? Based on the lessons of high-reliability science and past efforts to improve health care quality, it is believed that leadership commitment, full implementation of a safety culture, and thorough adoption of robust process improvement tools and methods together are the pathway most likely to lead to success. This approach offers the best hope yet for health care to achieve and sustain the elusive goal of consistent excellence in safety and quality.

Craig Clapper advises us to think of reliability as the platform for better patient care. "Reliability is the one thing that affects quality, safety and satisfaction well," he said. "By investing heavily in one thing, you can get three good families of outcomes." Clapper teaches High Reliability 2.0 for ACPE. The course is intended as follow-up to another ACPE course taught by Clapper, The Science of High Reliability. The introductory course lays a foundation, then High Reliability 2.0 gives participants the tools to take real-world solutions back to their organizations. Participants come away with nine practical skills:

1. Choosing appropriate reliability behaviors using aggregating analysis of harm events.

2. Implementing both a leader and a physician reliability bundle.

3. Building collaborative interactive teams (CITs).

4. Simplifying protocols by using human factors for written guidance documents.

5. Error-proofing an environment of care.

6. Increasing the reliability of checks and verification.

7. Using cause analysis methodology in peer review.

8. Quantifying the reliability of a time-out using probabilistic safety assessment (PSA).

9. Using reverse tracer methodology to measure process reliability.

No one in health care ever wants to hear about a serious clinical adverse event occurring, especially in his or her own hospital, but every clinician and caretaker knows that sometimes, despite best efforts, mistakes are made. Although there are plenty of guidelines to help hospitals avoid errors in the first place, there are few guidelines on what to do after the event, especially in terms of taking care of those involved.

The IHI, as part of its Innovation Series, has released a set of guidelines to help hospitals after an adverse event. The white paper, *Respectful Management of Serious Clinical Adverse Events*,[40] is designed to help organizations put a plan in place before an adverse event happens, similar to a fire evacuation plan or other emergency response. This plan should be simulated like any other contingency plan and should be based on previous adverse events while remaining adaptable to different kinds of events. It should also be revised and updated as appropriate.

The white paper says that hospitals have three main priorities during the aftermath of an adverse event: the patients and family, the frontline staff involved, and the organization as a whole, in that order. The paper's authors also suggest that hospitals create a crisis management team that can assemble immediately after adverse events. The team must focus on ensuring that the needs of patients, families, and staff members are met, while enhancing communication and support.

The hospital's first priority is the patient and family involved. A staff member should be available to them 24/7, and an apology should be issued when the hospital is at fault. The second priority is the frontline staff members who were involved in the incident. The IHI emphasizes a strong just culture, one that doesn't blame staff members, but rather supports them as "second victims" of the tragedy.The organization is the third priority; it must take steps to avoid the error in the future and communicate externally with regulatory agencies and media.

David Mayer, MD, and Timothy McDonald, MD, JD, University of Illinois Medical Center at Chicago, Ethics Forum participants, suggest steps that should be taken to encourage and support doctors in reporting adverse events to patients who have been harmed and their families.

Physicians strive to do no harm. Nonetheless, they seldom promise to disclose medical errors or mistakes that do harm to their patients. Disclosure is a professional responsibility that is desired by patients, endorsed by ethicists and professional organizations, and increasingly required by regulatory and government bodies. Although few now question the imperative to be honest and forthcoming following an injury, full disclosure communication with patients and families after an adverse event is still not the norm throughout the United States.

Full disclosure of a medical error is defined as a communication between a health care professional and a patient, family members or the patient's proxy that acknowledges the occurrence of an error, discusses what happened and describes the link between the error and outcomes in a manner that is meaningful to the patient.

Disclosure is based on the principle that all patients have a right to know the details associated with unexpected outcomes that occur during their care. Disclosure of medical errors and other relevant information after an unexpected adverse event provides opportunities for compassionate, professional and patient-centered care. It also allows for increased learning that could translate into safer systems-based practices and possible repair of patient-caregiver-health system trust.

Transparency and honesty begin with an organizational culture that openly reports adverse patient events, including near misses and unsafe conditions. The Joint Commission requires the establishment of a reporting system for adverse events by accredited organizations. Despite these mandates and perceived benefits of reporting, one survey of physicians in teaching hospitals revealed that only 54.8% of participating physicians knew how to report medical errors and only 39.5% knew what errors to report. Another survey found that only 31%

of interns or residents reported receiving instruction in error disclosure techniques.

The true value of transparency rests with the ability of organizations to rapidly investigate, analyze and learn from unanticipated outcomes. In addition to establishing whether an error caused the unanticipated outcome, the root cause analysis also can identify process breakdowns and opportunities to improve practices or individual performances. Identified potential process improvements should contain specific practice changes with measurable quality or safety indicators for long-term tracking of effectiveness. Those overseeing the investigation also are ideally situated to ensure that individuals involved with serious medical errors, the "second patients," receive emotional support and expert help following adverse events through care-for-the-caregiver programs. This requires personnel trained in process improvement, quality management and "second patient" issues to facilitate the team's inquiry. Transparency related to unexpected adverse outcomes, including full disclosure of medical errors, is central to the patient safety movement. Overall, disclosure programs implemented with a commitment to honesty and in a comprehensive manner with appropriate training and education should lead to reduced patient harm and improved processes, while engendering a safety culture in health care.

Even though more information about health care quality is available than ever before, few people use that information to make decisions about their care, or even ask doctors and nurses all the questions they have. The Robert Wood Johnson Foundation (RWJF) announced *Care About Your Care*, an effort in September 2011 to increase awareness about what consumers can do to identify and receive better health care.

"Questions Are the Answer," a new initiative from the U.S. Department of Health and Human Services' Agency for Healthcare Research and Quality (AHRQ) and the Ad Council, encourages clinicians and patients to engage in effective two-way communication to ensure safer care and better health outcomes.

People often fail to ask their doctors questions that could lead to fewer medical errors and better outcomes—and doctors don't routinely encourage them to do so. That's despite years of efforts to improve doctor-patient communication. Part of the problem is the intimidation factor that comes with the doctor's white coat. Also to blame are mounting time pressures that mean less physician or nurse interaction with patients, according to AHRQ. The agency is launching a new campaign to promote a solution that seems obvious but often doesn't happen: getting patients to ask questions. The aim is to get patients to prioritize their top concerns and questions before a medical encounter—and to get doctors to prompt patient questions in order to provide better care.

"Americans want more time with their doctors, but what hasn't sunk in is the importance of using the time you have with your doctor wisely," says Carolyn Clancy, the agency's director. For consumers, the agency is offering new online tools on its <u>website</u>, including an interactive "Question Builder." Patients talking to the doctor about a proposed surgery, for example, are prompted to ask how long it will take to recover. The site offers tips on what to do before, during, and after medical visits, such as calling the doctor if there are any side effects. Videos feature doctors discussing the importance of preparing for medical visits with a prioritized list of questions. Patients talk about how asking questions helped them get better care.

Also, the agency is launching its first ad campaign targeting doctors, with donated space in publications, including the *New England Journal of Medicine*, that reach two million clinicians. The ads urge doctors to ask patients about their health priorities, because "a simple question can reveal as much as a test." Doctors can also print or order free forms to help patients prioritize their top three questions.

An original series of new videos on the AHRQ Web site (<u>http://www.ahrq.gov/questions</u>) features real patients and clinicians discussing the importance of asking questions and sharing information. The Web site also features new resources to help patients to be prepared before, during, and after their medical appointments. The resources include: An interactive "Question Builder" tool that enables patients to create, prioritize, and print a personalized list of questions based on their health condition. A brochure, titled "Be More Involved in Your Health Care: Tips for Patients," offers helpful suggestions to follow before, during, and after a medical visit. Notepads help patients prioritize the top three questions they wish to address during their appointment.

The Lucian Leape Institute at the National Patient Safety Foundation (NPSF) released a paper outlining measures necessary in reforming and improving the safety of the health care system. The Institute's paper analyzes the proliferation of improvement efforts over the past decade, noting that progress toward improvement has been markedly slow. Some of this lack of progress, the report observes, may be attributed to the persistence of a medical ethos that discourages teamwork and transparency and undermines the establishment of accountability for safe care. The Lucian Leape Institute has identified five transforming concepts as fundamental to accelerating the work and making sustainable improvements in the safety of the health care system: full transparency, care integration, patient engagement, restoration of joy and meaning in work, and medical education reform.

So what do we need to change? The solution in the patient safety industry resides in *transformational* change. A great deal of work in patient safety and quality has historically been—and still is—incremental, not transformational. What if we could do something so transformational in patient safety and quality that it would produce the health care equivalent of Apple's stellar sales record: zero harm? What would it take? How would we redefine the standard of care and how care is delivered to the patient? I believe it will take a revamping of fortified cultures and an overhaul of safe system design.

Leaders in the quality and safety movement from all over the nation converged on the campus of Harvard University for the 10th Annual Quality Colloquium cosponsored by the Jefferson School of Population Health. Each year, Colloquium brings together national and international leaders in healthcare quality and safety. This year's focus was on patient safety and quality in light of healthcare reform.In the first morning of the program, three key leaders, including the CEO of the IHI in Boston, the National Patient Safety Foundation, and the AHRQ, set the tone for the rest of the week by challenging the audience to get further engaged in the movement. These leaders reminded us all that medical error remains the fourth leading cause of death in the U.S. and more must be done to protect our patients from harm. The research presentations covered a wide range of topics including the latest research on safety improvement in both the hospital and the office setting. Others presented an update on the role of hospital governance in quality and called for a renewed commitment on the part of board members to this agenda.

Diane Pinakiewicz, MBA, president of the National Patient Safety Foundation, spoke about accountability to patients for safe and effective care, emphasizing that providers need to focus on care from the view of the patient and work as a team to create the best patient experience possible. "There needs to be a culture of collective accountability-accountability to each other as well as the patients."

Communication and teamwork was also a common theme at the opening session. A lack of knowledge is clearly not the obstacle to quality health care, said Carolyn Clancy, MD, MPH, director of the Agency for Healthcare Research and Quality (AHRQ) in Washington, DC, who spoke on patient-centered system transformation and new opportunities for patient safety improvement. Rather, the problem is a lack of effective teamwork, she said. Simulation can be a powerful training tool toward working better as a team, said Clancy. Teamwork requires listening and communicating effectively, something health care providers do not do quite as well as those in other fields. Providers should be taught to communicate effectively with each other as well as with the patient.

Patient engagement is important, and most providers don't pay attention to it until it's needed, Pinakiewicz said. Trust, engagement, respect, and transparency are four necessary elements for accountability in health care, she noted.

Clancy championed the "three I's" as keys to finding these answers: information, incentives, and infrastructure. She highlighted the federal government's National Strategy for Quality Improvement in Healthcare, AHRQ's Effective Healthcare Program, the National Healthcare Quality and Disparities Reports, and the AHRQ Healthcare Innovations Exchange as valuable resources.

The second key, incentives, is up and coming. Clancy noted that the Centers for Medicare and Medicaid Innovation Patient Care Models—which includes patient care models such as Partnership for Patients and the Community-based Care Transition Program—provides many incentives for successful projects (http://*innovations.cms.gov*).

Last, a good infrastructure is necessary for improvement, said Clancy, stressing that quality improvement projects require an efficient system for collecting and reporting data. Electronic medical records, electronic prescribing, clinical decisions support, and personal health records are all components of a solid infrastructure, she noted. Providers need to be trained on how to use data correctly and effectively. She discussed Patient Safety Organizations (PSO), or groups that create a safe space to collect data on adverse events and create strategies to prevent them in the future. The data have federal guarantees of privilege and confidentiality. Clancy said PSOs are a new opportunity for patient safety improvement. So far, there are 81 PSOs in 30 states. AHRQ has worked to create what it calls "Common Formats" or common definitions of various adverse events so data can be more easily and correctly compared. They apply to:

- Incidents: patient safety events that reached the patient, regardless of whether there was actual patient harm.
- Near misses or close calls: patient safety events that did not reach the patient.
- Unsafe conditions: circumstances that increase the probability of a patient safety event

AHRQ plans to use the data in a network to gather national and regional statistics.

Wachter and Pronovost suggest that the urgency of the task also demands that we stop averting our eyes from the need to balance "no blame" and accountability.[37] "No blame" is not a moral imperative—and even if it seems that way to providers, it most definitely does not to patients and their advocates. Rather, it is a tactic to help us achieve ends (safe and high-quality care) for which we will, quite appropriately, be held accountable. Said another way, "no blame" is a tool, and often an extraordinarily useful one. But for some mature patient-safety practices, it is simply the wrong tool. Finding this balance will be challenging. One must recognize that reasonable people will differ on many of the details and that individual organizations may need customized approaches. The goal is simply to promote conversations and meaningful action. It is time to raise this topic to the top of our agenda. Moreover, clinicians must learn accountability for patient outcomes for which there is limited empirical evidence. Ultimately, physicians must be held accountable for their clinical behaviors, and their leaders must accept the responsibilities to lead these efforts.

Most health care providers embraced the "no blame" model as a refreshing change from an errors landscape previously dominated by a malpractice system that was generally judged as punitive and arbitrary. In 1988, Dr. Arnold Relman, editor of the *New England Journal of Medicine*, wrote that the U.S. had seen two revolutions in the medical care system since WW II. He predicted that we were on the threshold of a third related to assessment and accountability.[38]

Accountability in medicine, once assigned primarily to individual doctors, is today increasingly shared by groups of health-care providers.[39-40] Because patient safety experts emphasize that most errors are caused not by individual providers, but rather by system breakdowns in complex health-care teams, individual doctors are left to wonder where their accountability lies. Increasingly, teams deliver care. But patients and doctors alike still think of accountability in individual terms, and the law often measures it that way. We discuss "collective accountability," suggesting that this construct may offer a way to balance a "just culture" and a doctor's specific responsibilities within the framework of team delivery of care. The concept of collective accountability requires doctors to adopt transparent behaviors, learn new skills for improving team performance, and participate in institutional safety initiatives to evaluate errors and implement plans for preventing recurrences. It also means that institutions need to prioritize team training, develop robust, non-punitive reporting systems, support clinicians after adverse events and medical error, and develop ways to compensate patients who are harmed by errors.

A conceptual leap to collective accountability may help overcome long-standing professional and societal norms that not only reinforce individual blame and impede patient safety but may also leave the patient and family without a true advocate. So, as we conclude this chapter, on progress, or lack of it, in establishing a comprehensive patient safety movement, we turn again to the requirements:

We have established a clear consensus: To arrive at health care that is high quality—that is, safe, effective, patient-centered, efficient, delivered on a timely basis, and devoid of disparities based on race or ethnicity. The medical profession must endorse the concept that the public has a right to expect health care that is safe and effective. The profession is responsible to individual patients and to the public to continuously seek to improve the quality of medical care and make sure that health care services are provided as safely as possible.

Health care organizations should strive to become high-reliability systems displaying consistent performance at high levels of safety over long periods. Several common key features facilitate the maintenance of consistent excellence. These features incorporate a "collective mindfulness," which is a dominant attitude, or cultural feature, that all high-reliability organizations display. Collective accountability and transparency must be essential features. In addition, remember the three critical changes that health care must make to become a high-reliability industry:

1. The responsibility of leadership to make high reliability the priority.
2. The importance of creating a culture of safety within an organization.
3. The use of proven quality methods—Lean Six Sigma and change management (known together as robust process improvement™)—to systematically improve processes and avoid common, crucial failures.

So what do we need to change? The solution in the patient safety industry resides in *transformational* change The Lucian Leape Institute has identified transforming concepts as fundamental. Moreover, *the* need to balance "no blame" and accountability will be challenging. Clinicians must learn accountability for patient outcomes for which there is limited empirical evidence. Ultimately, physicians must be held accountable for their clinical behaviors, and their leaders must accept the responsibilities to lead these efforts.

References

1. Institute of Medicine. *To Err Is Human: Building a Safe Health System.* Washington D.C.: National Academy Press, 1999.

2. Schimmel, E.M. "The hazards of hospitalization." Annals of Internal Medicine. 60:100-10, 1964.

3. Wachter, R.M. "Patient Safety At Ten: Unmistakable Progress, Troubling Gaps," http://hospitalmedicine.ucsf.edu/downloads/patient_safety_at_ten.pdf.

4. Institute of Medicine. *Crossing the Quality Chasm: A New Health System for the 21st Century.* Washington D.C.: National Academy Press, 2001.

5. Berwick,D.M. A User's Manual for the "IOM's Quality Chasm Report." *Health Affairs*, 2002:21(3):80-90, May-June 2002.

6. Dentzer, S. "Still Crossing The Quality Chasm—Or Suspended Over It?" *Health Affairs* 30(4):554-5, April 30, 2011.

7. "Designing Consumer Reporting Systems for Patient Safety", http://ahrq.gov/qual/consreporting/.

8. *Closing the Quality Gap: Revisiting the State of the Science:Series Overview.* Rockville, MD, April 2011. http://www.ahrq.gov/clinic/tp/gapprevor.htm

9. Jiang, J., and others. "Board Oversight of Quality: Any Difference in Process Care and Mortality." Journal of Health Care Management 54(1):15-30, Jan./Feb. 2009.

10. "Leaders Media Intelligence Report: The Drive to Patient Safety." May 2011, http://content.hcpro.com/pdf/content/266092.pdf.

11. Chen, P.W. "A Better Way to Keep Patients Safe." *New York Times*, Aug. 4, 2011.

12. "American College of Surgeons announces National Surgical Quality Improvement Program. *Patient Safety Monitor Alert*, August 3, 2011.

13. Pronovost, P.J., and Freischlag, J.A. "Improving Teamwork to Reduce Surgical Mortality." JAMA 304(15):1721-2, Oct. 20,2010.

14. Haynes, A.B., and others "A Surgical Safety Checklist to Reduce Morbidity and Mortality in a Global Population." *New England Journal of Medicine* 360(5):491-499, Jan. 29, 2009.

15. Hall, B.L., and others. "Does Surgical Quality Improve in the American College of Surgeons. National Surgical Quality Improvement Program." Annals of Surgery 250(3):363-76, Sept. 2009.

16. Ali, M., and others. "Preoperative Surgical Briefings Do Not Delay Operating Room Start Times and Are Popular With Surgical Team Members." *Journal of Patient Safety* 7(3):139-43, Sept. 2011.

17. Birkmeyer, J.D. "Strategies for Improving Surgical Quality—Checklists and Beyond." *New England Journal of Medicine* 363(20):1963-5, November 11, 2010.

18. "Joint Commission Addresses Wrong-site Surgery. Pilot organizations Discuss Their Experiences." *Patient Safety Monitor*, Sept. 1, 2011.

19. Stulberg, J.J., and others. "Adherence to Surgical Care Improvement Project Measures and the Association with Postoperative Infections.: *JAMA* 303(24):2479-85, June 23, 2010.

20. Muller, M.P., and Detsky, A.S. "Public Reporting of Hospital Hand Hygiene Compliance—Helpful or Harmful?" *JAMA* 304(10):1116-1117, Sept. 8, 2010.

21. Kahn, J.M., and Angus, D.C. "Going Home on the Right Medications: Prescription Errors and Transitions of Care." *JAMA*. 306(8):878-879, Aug. 24, 2011.

22. DeWalt, D.A. "Ensuring Safe and Effective Use of Medication and Health Care: Perfecting the Dismount." *JAMA*. 304(23):2641-2, Dec 15, 2010.

23. Kahn, J.M., and Angus, D.C. "Prescription Errors and Transitions of Care. 10th Annual Quality Colloquium co sponsored by the Jefferson School of Population Health.

24. Moore, P. "Medicines Reconciliation Using a Shared Electronic Health Care Record." *Journal of Patient* Safety 7(3): 148-54,

25. Kuehn, B. M. "Bar Codes Improve Safety." *JAMA* 303(24):2464, June 23-30, 2010.

26. Kilo, C.M., and Larson, E.B. "Exploring the Harmful Effects of Health Care." *JAMA* 302(1):89-91, July 1, 2009.

27. "Eliminating Preventable Harm by Defining It." *Patient Safety Monitor*, March 1, 2011.

28. Cors, W.K., and Sagin, T. "Overtreatment in Health Care: How Much Is Too Much." *Physician Executive Journal* 37(5):10-6, Sept.-Oct, 2011.

29. Einstein, A.J. "Radiation Protection of Patients Undergoing Cardiac Computed Tomographic Angiography." *JAMA* 301(5):545-547, Feb. 4, 2009.

30. Rumsfeld, J.S., and Peterson, E.D. "Achieving Meaningful Device Surveillance from Reaction to Proaction." *JAMA*.304(18):2065-6, Nov. 10, 2010.

31. Newman-Toker, D.E., and Pronovost, P.J. "Diagnostic Errors—The Next Frontier for Patient Safety." *JAMA* 301(10):1060-2, Mar. 11, 2009.

32. Sax, H., and others. "Can Aviation-based Team Training Elicit Sustainable Behavioral Change?" *Archives of Surgery* 144(12):1133-7, Dec. 2009.

33. Helkind, S.J., Sinnett, J.C. "Patient Care, Square-Rigger Sailing, and Safety." *JAMA* 300(14):1691-3, Oct. 8, 2008.

34. Reason, J.T. *Human Error*. New York: Cambridge University Press, 1990.

35. Reason, J. "Human Error: Models and Management." *British Medical Journal* 320(7237):771-3, March 18, 2000.

36. Chassin, M.R., and Loeb, J. "The Ongoing Quality Improvement Journey: Next Stop, High Reliability." 30(4):559-68, April 14, 2011.

37. Wachter, R.M., and Pronovost, P.J. "Balancing "No Blame" with Accountability in Patient Safety." *New England Journal of Medicine* 361(14):1401-6, Oct. 1, 2009.

38. Relman, A.S. "Assessment and Accountability: The Third Revolution in Medical Care." *New England Journal of Medicine* 319(18):1220–2, Nov. 3, 1988.

39. Pronovost, P.J. "Learning Accountability for Patient Outcomes." *JAMA* 304(2):204-5, July 14, 2010.

40. Bell, S.K., and others. "Accountability for Medical Error: Moving Beyond Blame to Advocacy. *Chest* 2011 Aug;140(2):519-26, Aug. 2011.

Important Safety Web Resources

Centers for Disease Control and Prevention: www.cdc.gov
Environmental Protection Agency: www.epa.gov
Nuclear Regulatory Commission: www.nrc.gov
U.S. Office of Hazardous Materials Safety: hazmat.dot.gov
Hospitals for a Healthy Environment: www.h2e-online.org/
Federal Register: www.access.gpo.gov
Food and Drug Administration: www.fda.gov
OSHA: www.osha.gov
National Institute for Occupational Safety and Health: www.cdc.gov
The Joint Commission: www.jointcommission.org
National Fire Protection Association: www.nfpa.org
American Society for Healthcare Engineering: www.ashe.org
Centers for Medicare & Medicaid Services: www.cms.hss.gov
American Institute of Architects: www.aia.org
www.facs.org/quality.
www.qualityforum.org
IOM.org
www.patientsafety.gov
www.npsf.org/
www.nlm.nih.gov/medlineplus/patientsafety.html
www.patientsafety.org/
www.aha.org/advocacy-issues/quality/index.shtml
www.anesthesiapatientsafety.com
www.medscape.com/resource/patientsafety
www.asahq.org
www.ccforpatientsafety.org
www.leapfroggroup.org
www.p4ps.org
www.projectpatientcare.org
psnet.ahrq.gov

Chapter 8

Health Law Overview

by Henry Casale, JD and Susan Lapenta, JD

Health law changes constantly. In some cases, such as with telemedicine, these changes are dictated by advances in technology that require the law to "catch up" with industry practice. In other cases, such as with Medicare reimbursement for particular services, changes in the law reflect a conscious decision by the government to influence the behavior of health care providers in a certain manner.

This chapter examines the development of the law in the following areas: legal theories used by injured patients to sue health care entities, protection available to participants in the peer review process, regulations implementing the privacy provisions of the Health Insurance Portability and Accountability Act ("HIPAA"), "on-call" provisions of the Emergency Medical Treatment and Active Labor Act ("EMTALA"), the Medicare anti-kickback law, the Stark law, and the Patient Protection and Affordable Care Act (the "Health Reform Law"). The discussion provides a snapshot of these areas at this particular time. Keep in mind that the law is not static (especially in health care) and that these laws will likely change with time.

Trends in Liability

Several major theories have been used by injured patients to sue health care entities such as hospitals, managed care organizations and physician groups, including the doctrine of respondeat superior, the doctrine of ostensible agency or "holding out," and negligent credentialing.

Respondeat Superior

Under the doctrine of respondeat superior, an employer or supervisor is held liable for the negligent acts of its employees. While this legal doctrine is based in part on the employer's actual control or right to control the activities of its employees, it also reflects a traditional social policy that places the risk of losses caused by negligent conduct of employees on employers as a cost of doing business. Additionally, this doctrine focuses on compensating the victims of employees' negligent acts by placing liability on the party with the "deeper pockets." It is important to note that the doctrine does not absolve the employee of responsibility for negligent conduct; it merely allows the injured patient to sue the employer and increases the likelihood of recovery.

Ostensible Agency

Even after the application of the doctrine of respondeat superior in the health care field, injured patients often still did not have a right to sue hospitals when injuries were caused by physicians. Most physicians are independent contractors of hospitals, not employees, and hospitals were not liable for their actions. But creative lawyers thought up another way to include hospitals in malpractice suits, which became known as the doctrine of ostensible agency (sometimes called "apparent agency") or the "holding out" doctrine.

Almost all early ostensible agency or "holding out" cases involved patients who had come to hospital emergency departments and had suffered injuries at the hands of either emergency department physicians or on-call physicians. The argument was that these physicians were selected by the hospitals and/or appeared to be employees or agents of the hospitals, and thus the hospitals should be held responsible for the physicians' negligent acts. For the most part, the courts have agreed with this theory and allowed these claims to go forward against hospitals. In addition, the theory has been expanded beyond emergency departments and hospitals to the managed care arena.

Negligent Credentialing

In recent years, public demand for professional accountability has had a great influence on credentialing activities. Hospital boards are also being pressured by accrediting organizations, state and federal regulators, and the general public to make certain that clinical privileges are based on measured performance.

Laws governing the credentialing process are derived from many sources, including state licensure statutes, the Medicare Conditions of Participation, and case law. In addition, the standards developed by hospital accrediting bodies–The Joint Commission, the Healthcare Facilities and Accreditation Program ("HFAP"), and DNV Healthcare–are particularly important. Although accreditation standards do not rise to the level of statutes or governmental regulations, courts frequently defer to them as evidence of the appropriate standard of care.

These sources of law impose on the governing body the duty to assess the qualifications and ongoing capabilities of those who perform clinical services in the hospital. It is the governing body of the hospital that is ultimately responsible for care rendered to hospital patients and that then revocably delegates this responsibility to the organized medical staff.

Health care entities that fail in their duty to assess the qualifications of physicians can be found liable under the doctrine of corporate liability for negligent credentialing. This doctrine, which is increasingly gaining judicial acceptance, holds health care entities liable for failing to have systems in place that adequately assess and ensure high-quality patient care. Health care entities now clearly have the legal duty to monitor the activities of professionals who practice in their facilities or are affiliated with them. Failure to initiate corrective action when necessary and appropriate can lead to a finding of liability.

Peer Review Protection

Health Care Quality Improvement Act

A number of legal protections are available to hospitals, HMOs, and group practices that engage in peer review activities. The most significant of these is the Health Care Quality Improvement Act of 1986 (HCQIA).

HCQIA was designed to encourage the performance of peer review activity and, in certain cases, the use of the results of peer review by other hospitals and licensing authorities. An underlying assumption in the law is that individuals will be more candid in providing information and more willing to take needed action if the threat of liability is removed or reduced. Thus, HCQIA generally shields individuals from liability for their performance of peer review activities.

HCQIA provides two different types of immunity. There is immunity for individuals who provide information to peer review bodies. There is also immunity for the peer reviewers themselves.

The immunity for individuals who provide information is very broad. HCQIA states that any person who provides information to a professional review body regarding the competence or professional conduct of a physician shall be immune from liability and damages under any federal or state law unless the information provided is false and the person providing it knew that it was false.

Professional review bodies and other persons who assist them in professional review activities are also protected from damage suits as long as the professional review was taken in the reasonable belief that the action was in the furtherance of high-quality health care, after a reasonable effort to obtain the facts of the matter, after adequate notice and hearing procedures are afforded to the physician involved, and in the reasonable belief that the action was warranted by the facts known.

As long as these standards are met, the health care entity, and the individuals involved in its professional review activities, will be immune from damages. HCQIA also provides additional protection by allowing defendants in suits challenging professional review actions to recover attorneys' fees and the costs of defense in the event that they substantially prevail in the action.

The immunity provided for professional review activities is not absolute. The immunity does not apply to actions brought under the federal civil rights laws, injunction or declaratory judgment actions, actions by governmental agencies such as the Federal Trade Commission, or criminal proceedings. The immunity also does not apply to actions brought by nonphysician practitioners, such as podiatrists or chiropractors.

State Law Protections

The important role of peer review committees in improving patient care has been recognized by state legislatures, Congress, and the courts. Virtually every state legislature has enacted a "peer review" statute. Like the HCQIA, these statutes protect individuals involved in the peer review process from liability. Often state peer review statutes provide qualified immunity. This means that immunity is available if the party acts in "good faith" or "without malice." These standards are subjective and thus courts are sometimes unwilling to dismiss a claim unless and until a jury has determined there has been no malice. However, the state peer review statutes protect peer review documents from discovery and admissibility in lawsuits; something HCQIA does not do.

Patient Safety and Quality Improvement Act

The Patient Safety and Quality Improvement Act is another potential source of protection for peer review documents. The law allows for the creation of Patient Safety Organizations (PSOs). Providers can submit their quality information to a PSO. PSOs will aggregate and analyze these data and then report them back to providers in order to improve patient outcomes and promote a "culture of safety." The information that is (i) assembled or developed for reporting to the PSO, (ii) developed by the PSO for the conduct of patient safety activities, and (iii) constitutes the deliberations or analysis of, or identifies the fact of reporting to, a patient safety evaluation system will all be privileged as "Patient Safety Work Product" and is protected from discovery.

Other Protections

Other protections available to physicians who are involved in the peer review process include the release and immunity language that is found in most applications signed by physicians seeking appointment to a hospital's medical staff or appointment to a managed care organization's provider panel. In several cases courts have dismissed claims based on that language. Similar language may appear in bylaws and can also be used as a shield against liability.

Another important source of protection is in the health care entity's directors' and officers' (D & O) insurance policy. This protection is available for physicians who carry out peer review functions on behalf of the health care entity. In most instances, the D & O insurance covers the cost of defense as well as the cost of any award in the off chance that there is one.

A health care entity's indemnification policy is yet another source of protection. Most corporate bylaws include an indemnification provision to protect members of the board, administration, and others who perform functions on behalf of the organization. Peer review is just one function that would be protected by the indemnification clause.

In all of these protections, however, it is imperative that the physician be functioning on behalf of a health care entity. To the extent that a physician was operating in his or her personal capacity, the protection would be lost and individual liability could occur.

HIPAA

"HIPAA," which stands for "Health Insurance Portability and Accountability Act," is a federal law that governs many aspects of health care. These days, most people use the term HIPAA to refer to the privacy and security regulations that govern the manner in which physicians, hospitals, health plans, and other "covered entities" use, disclose, and protect a patient's health information. Ironically, the HIPAA Privacy Rule grew out of an attempt to reduce the burden of administering health care claims by requiring providers and payers to standardize the manner in which they coded and processed claims. The privacy and security features of the law were incidental to that primary goal. Many feared that the increased use of electronic transactions would increase the risk that identifiable health information would be improperly disclosed. As a result, the Health Insurance Portability and Accountability Act, approved by Congress in 1996, included restrictions on the ways that health information can be used and disclosed, as well as specific requirements governing how covered entities secure health information in their possession. HIPAA was amended by the HITECH (Health Information Technology for Economic and

Clinical Health) Act to provide additional protections for patients and health plan beneficiaries. For example, the breach notification regulations were passed as part of HITECH, requiring covered entities to notify individuals when certain "breaches" of their health information occur.

Who Is Covered by HIPAA?

The HIPAA Privacy Rule applies to "covered entities" and their "business associates." The term "covered entity" includes all health plans and "health care clearinghouses" (generally, entities that provide coding services), along with health care providers who transmit "protected health information" ("PHI") as part of a standard transaction in electronic form.

"Protected health information" is a term of art, with a long regulatory definition. But generally, PHI is any information about the identity or health of a patient or health plan enrollee. This includes some surprising information. For example, identifying information would include the serial number on any device implanted into a patient.

As already mentioned, the transmission of PHI in electronic form is a key criterion in determining whether a health care provider is a covered entity. Be clear, however, that once an entity qualifies as a covered entity, the Privacy Rule requires it to protect all forms of PHI: electronic, "hard copy" (paper records, film, etc.), and oral communications. The Security Rule, on the other hand, applies only to PHI in electronic form.

Privacy Rule

The privacy regulations address three topics: uses and disclosures of health information, patient rights with respect to their own health information, and administrative issues.

Uses and Disclosures of Health Information

The manner in which the Privacy Rule restricts a physician's use or disclosure of PHI can be broken into three categories.

- Physicians may make certain uses and disclosures without obtaining the patient's authorization and without giving the patient an opportunity to object.
- Physicians may make other uses and disclosures without obtaining a patient's written authorization, but only after giving the patient an opportunity to object to the use or disclosure.
- All other disclosures require a patient's written authorization.

No Patient Authorization Required

Physicians may use or disclose PHI for three broad purposes without patient authorization: treatment, payment, and health care operations. For example, under the Privacy Rule, a primary care physician may send a patient's medical record without patient authorization to a specialist who will treat the patient. Likewise, a physician may disclose PHI directly to a health plan for the purpose of obtaining payment for services provided or may disclose PHI to another health care provider to enable it to bill for its services. The HITECH rule creates one exception. If the patient pays up front for a service and asks that a physician not tell his or her health plan about that service, then the physician must comply with the request. "Health care operations" is a catch-all term that allows physicians to use or disclose PHI for activities related to their general management and administration, including quality assessment and improvement, credentialing, legal services, and licensing.

The Privacy Rule also permits physicians to use or disclose PHI without patient authorization for a number of enumerated purposes. Generally, these purposes involve public health, public safety, or some other important public concern. Thus, PHI may be used or disclosed without patient authorization when required by law; for public health purposes; in cases dealing with victims of abuse; for health oversight or law enforcement purposes; in the course of judicial or administrative proceedings; when dealing with decedents, cadavers, or tissue donation; for certain research purposes; when necessary to avert serious threat to health or safety; and for specialized government functions.

Patient Opportunity to Object

Other uses and disclosures can be made without patient authorization, but only after the patient has been given an opportunity to object. This opportunity to object need not be in writing. For example, a physician may simply ask if the patient objects to any of the uses and disclosures. Or, in some cases, the physician may presume that the patient does not object (for example, the patient sends her husband to the doctor's office to pick up a prescription sample and the husband mentions the patient by name and the fact that he is picking up the sample on her behalf).

Two disclosures in this category are particularly relevant to physicians. First, the Privacy Rule states that physicians may disclose information to family members, friends, or other individuals who are involved in the patient's care. In this case, the information disclosed is limited to that which is directly relevant to the person's involvement in the patient's care. Second, the Privacy Rule states that physicians may disclose a patient's health information to notify family members of a patient's condition.

However, the only information that may be disclosed for notification purposes is the patient's location and general condition. Thus, if a physician wishes to provide detailed information of a patient's condition to family members, and the family members are *not* involved in the patient's care, the physician must first obtain the patient's written authorization.

This restriction on a physician's ability to communicate with family members who are not involved in the patient's care has caused a great deal of concern and frustration in the medical community. For example, physicians argue that relatives from out of state who are not involved in the patient's care should be permitted to receive more information than simply the patient's location or general condition and that the Privacy Rule interferes with family relations. However, the federal government has chosen to protect the individual's right to control his or her own health information over any rights that family members may assert.

Patient Authorization Required

Written authorization from the patient is required for all uses and disclosures of PHI that are not specifically permitted by the regulations. The Privacy Rule requires that numerous specific elements be included in every such authorization form, including a description of the information in question, the persons authorized to disclose or receive the information, the purpose of the disclosure, the signature of the individual, and a description of the various rights of the patient. Because the requirements for authorization forms are quite numerous and complicated, it is wise for each physician or group practice to have a patient sign his or her own authorization form prior to disclosing any records (rather than relying on an authorization form provided by a third party, already signed by the patient).

"Minimum Necessary" Rule

Covered entities are required to make a reasonable effort to limit their use or disclosure of PHI to the "minimum necessary" to accomplish the intended purpose of the use or disclosure. The purpose of this requirement is to prevent disclosure of all information relating to a patient when only a few items of information are necessary. The minimum necessary standard applies both to the disclosure of PHI to outside entities and to uses of PHI internally, at a physician's office.

There are several significant exceptions to the minimum necessary rule. Most important, the rule does *not* apply to disclosures to health care providers for treatment purposes. The federal government recognized that health care providers involved in the care of the patient should have access to the entire medical record. However, personnel who are not involved in the care of the patient should have access only to PHI that is necessary for them to perform their duties.

Since the original passage of the privacy regulations, critics have argued that the minimum necessary rule is too broad and provides covered entities with too much discretion to determine how much PHI to use or disclose. Accordingly, the Department of Health and Human Services is in the process of reconsidering the minimum necessary standard and providing more stringent restrictions in this area.

Incidental Disclosures of PHI

The Privacy Rule recognizes that disclosures that are incidental to an otherwise permitted use or disclosure may occur. For example, a visitor to a physician's office may overhear a conversation between a physician and a nurse about another patient or may observe the names of other patients while signing in at the physician's office. Such incidental disclosures are not considered violations of the Privacy Rule as long as the physician has taken "reasonable safeguards" to prevent the disclosure. For example, a physician might isolate filing cabinets or records rooms, require passwords to access computers containing PHI, or add curtains to areas where oral communications often occur between physicians and patients. The safeguards that are "reasonable" will vary with the size of the covered entity, its resources, the nature of the PHI, and the effect of the safeguard on patient care.

Disclosures to Business Associates

A "business associate" is an entity that makes use of PHI to perform a function on behalf of or to provide a service (generally, an administrative service, such as legal services) to a covered entity. The Privacy Rule requires covered entities to enter into agreements with their business associates to ensure that the business associates appropriately safeguard the PHI they receive from the covered entity. In addition, the HITECH rule modified HIPAA to apply directly to business associates. Accordingly, business associates may now be directly responsible to the government for violations of the privacy and security rules.

Patient Rights

In addition to restricting the way PHI is used and disclosed, the HIPAA privacy rule gave patients new rights to control their health information. Physicians must provide every patient with a "Notice of Privacy Practices," and they must make a good faith effort to obtain the patient's written acknowledgment that he or she received the notice. The notice must inform patients of their rights and the physician's duties with respect to PHI, as well as the covered entity's procedures to protect the privacy of PHI and to comply with the Privacy Rule.

Health care providers who have direct treatment relationships with patients are required to provide the notice no later than the date of the first delivery of service. They must also post the notice in a clear and prominent location. If the provider maintains a website, the notice must be posted there as well. A good faith effort must be made to obtain written acknowledgment of receipt of the notice only at the time of the first delivery of service. It is not required at every visit or patient encounter.

The Privacy Rule also gives patients the rights to request restrictions on the uses and disclosures of their PHI, gain access to their PHI, request amendment to their PHI, and obtain an accounting of the manner in which their PHI has been disclosed by a covered entity.

Preemption of State Law

The Privacy Rule "preempts," or overrides, any state laws that conflict with it, unless the state laws are more protective of patients' rights. In other words, the Privacy Rule creates a "floor" by establishing a certain minimum level of privacy protection. If state law provides greater privacy protection, it must be followed.

The preemption provision receives very little attention, but it creates more complexity than any other provision of the Privacy Rule. It is not enough for physicians to understand only the Privacy Rule. They must become familiar with both the Privacy Rule and the numerous state laws (which are found in a variety of sources, including state statutes, regulations, and judicial decisions) that address patient privacy. Physicians must then compare the two and follow the law that is more protective of privacy. It is very common for states to have laws that are more protective of HIV and AIDS-related information, mental health records, drug and alcohol records, and genetic testing.

Security Rule

By way of background, the HIPAA Security Rule requires physicians to "[e]nsure the confidentiality, integrity, and availability of all electronic protected health information the covered entity creates, receives, maintains, or transmits." The Rule gives hospitals a great deal of flexibility in meeting this requirement. It does not prescribe the use of specific technologies (recognizing the rapid pace at which technology is changing) and does not impose detailed requirements for policies that should be used to protect electronic health information.

The Security Rule's provisions are numerous and detailed, and all covered entities would be well advised to consult not only with their legal counsel regarding compliance, but also with the providers of IT for the physician's practice. Among other things that physician practices should consider in complying with the Security Rule are the following:

1. Requiring a username and password for access to electronic PHI.

2. Automatic log-outs on computers that contain PHI after a specified period.

3. Keeping a written record of all hardware that contains PHI (for example, laptops, iPads, iPhones) to ensure that all are password-protected, accounted for, and erased before being sold or discarded—or whenever the employee who owns the hardware terminates employment.

4. Maintaining firewalls and anti-viral software to protect medical records from external hacking.

5. Utilizing a medical record system that tracks access (and performing routine audits of access to ensure employees are viewing records only for work-related purposes).

Depending on the size of a physician practice and the resources available to it, more or less may be necessary to secure electronic PHI. What is most important is that physicians are aware of the Security Rule and the need to comply and that they take steps to do so. Because the Security Rule is so complicated and because it followed the privacy regulations by a couple of years, it received less fanfare. Compliance with the security regulations has been varied, although it has been improving in recent years as more and more physician practices move to electronic health records systems (which usually have security features built in).

Breach Notification Regulations

As noted above, the HITECH Act of 2009 made significant changes to the HIPAA Privacy and Security Rules. One of the most important revisions is a requirement that covered entities notify a patient if there is a breach of "unsecured" PHI related to that patient. Regulations implementing the breach notification provisions were passed on August 24, 2009.

The breach notification requirements apply only to PHI that is unsecured. Thus, if PHI has been "secured," hospitals have no obligation to notify patients of a breach of that information. The Department of Health and Human Services has provided very detailed information regarding what constitutes "secured" PHI. Essentially, the guidance requires that PHI be encrypted (for electronic PHI) or be properly destroyed (for paper or hard copy PHI) in order to be "secured."

If unsecured information is breached—and the covered entity determines that harm to the patient's reputation or finances is likely—the patient must be notified about the breach. And at the end of each year, the covered entity must notify the Department of Health and Human Services of all breach notifications it made that year. If the breach involves more than 500 patients from the same state, additional steps are required, such as notification of the media and immediate reporting to the Department.

Conclusion

It is easy to be overwhelmed by the size and complexity of the Privacy and Security Rules. The regulations, their governmental interpretations and whitepapers, and subsequent revisions span thousands of pages in the *Federal Register*! We can confidently report that in the near decade since the rules were passed, awareness of patient confidentiality and sensitivity within the health care industry to the importance of confidentiality has increased. Likewise, spending on IT that secures patient health information has increased, and electronic medical records are undoubtedly better protected from hacking and theft. This is good news, because the Department of Health and Human Services recently declared that the honeymoon phase of HIPAA implementation is over and enforcement activities (including some of the first fines, settlements, and criminal convictions) have begun.

EMTALA

The Emergency Medical Treatment and Active Labor Act (EMTALA) was one of the first patient safety statutes. It was designed to make sure that hospitals did not deny care to patients in an emergency condition. EMTALA requires that hospitals with an emergency department provide a medical screening examination for any individual who presents seeking care or treatment. If a determination is made that the patient has an emergency medical condition, the hospital must provide stabilizing treatment. EMTALA also provides rules concerning how and when the patient may be transferred if the hospital is unable to treat the individual because it lacks the capability or facility to treat the patient..

On-Call Requirements

EMTALA's requirement that patients be provided with stabilizing treatment is the basis for the on-call list that hospitals are required by law to maintain. The Centers for Medicare and Medicaid Services (CMS), the federal agency that administers EMTALA, has stated that "[t]he purpose of the on-call list is to ensure that the emergency department is prospectively aware of which physicians, including specialists and subspecialists, are available to provide treatment necessary to stabilize individuals with emergency medical conditions. If a hospital offers a service to the public, the service should be available through on-call coverage of the emergency department."

On-call physicians who fail to respond to a call request are subject to a fine of up to $50,000 and exclusion from Medicare. Moreover, EMTALA has a built-in mechanism for ensuring that the pertinent federal agencies learn of any patient transfer caused by the refusal of the scheduled on-call physician to respond to call. When any transfer occurs under EMTALA, the patient's medical record must be sent along with the patient. That medical record must contain "the name and address of any on-call physician...who has refused or failed to appear within a reasonable time to provide necessary stabilizing treatment." The hospital that receives the patient is required to report that violation to the federal government or risk being in violation of EMTALA itself.

EMTALA's requirement that hospitals maintain a call list and that physicians respond when called raises a difficult question: How often must a physician serve on call? This issue is particularly troubling when a hospital's medical staff includes only one or two physicians in a given specialty. Until May 9, 2002, this question was generally answered by the "three-physician rule." This was an informal, unpublished rule used by CMS that required hospitals with three physician specialists on the medical staff to provide call coverage in that specialty 24 hours a day, 365 days a year. By application of the three-physician rule, physicians would generally not be expected to provide more than 10 days of call coverage per month.

CMS has subsequently disavowed the three-physician rule. Instead, CMS will apply the "all relevant factors" test. Relevant factors include the number of physicians on staff, other demands on these physicians, and the frequency with which the hospital's patients typically require services of on-call physicians in a particular specialty.

Anti-Kickback Statute

The anti-kickback statute makes it a criminal offense to knowingly and willfully offer, pay, solicit, or receive any remuneration to induce referrals of items or services reimbursable by any federal health care program. The statute ascribes criminal liability to parties on both sides of an impermissible "kickback" transaction. For purposes of the anti-kickback statute, "remuneration" includes the transfer of anything of value, in cash or in kind, directly or indirectly, covertly or overtly. The statute has been interpreted to cover any arrangement in which one purpose of the remuneration is to obtain money for the referral of services or to induce further referrals. As will be discussed below, the Anti-Kickback statute may also be enforced by the Office of Inspector General of HHS (the "OIG") in an administrative proceeding.

The federal Department of Health and Human Services has issued regulations identifying business practices that do not constitute a violation of the anti-kickback statute. These "safe harbors" are voluntary and must be fully complied with in order to apply. There are safe harbors for investment interests, space leases, equipment rental, personal services contracts, sales of a physician's practice, referral arrangements, and other activities, as long as the specific requirements set forth in the regulation are satisfied. By statute employment agreements are exempt from the anti-kickback statute.

Violation of the anti-kickback statute constitutes a felony punishable by a maximum fine of $25,000, imprisonment of up to five years, or both. Conviction will also lead to automatic exclusion from federal health care programs, including Medicare and Medicaid. The OIG can also initiate administrative proceedings to exclude persons from federal and state health care programs and/or to impose civil monetary penalties. Claims submitted to Medicare as a result of the unlawful arrangement may also be considered to be false claims under the federal False Claims Act and subject to the liability described below.

The federal government's interpretation of the anti-kickback statute continually evolves, formally through case law and informally through the use of compliance guidance, "fraud alerts," and "advisory opinions." The courts have found that arrangements such as rent or services at other than fair market value will violate the anti-kickback statute if the government can prove that at least one purpose of the remuneration was to induce the referral of patients or services that are paid for in whole or in part by a federal health care program (U.S. v. Greber, 760 F.2d 68 (3rd Cir.) *cert. denied*, 474 U.S. 988 (1985). However, the fact that the government must prove an unlawful intent makes the enforcement of this statute extremely fact-specific.

Compliance guidance and fraud alerts highlight significant concerns identified by the government, while advisory opinions respond to requests for guidance by health care providers with respect to specific factual situations. Although this informal guidance does not have the force of law, it does indicate the government's approach at any given time to enforcement of the anti-kickback statute.

Stark Law

In his introductory remarks to the Comprehensive Physician Ownership and Referral Act of 1993, Congressman Stark stated that "the only way to protect health care consumers from unnecessary referrals is to impose a bright line rule." In order to accomplish this intent, Section 1877 of the Social Security Act, also known as the "Stark Law": (1) prohibits a physician from making referrals for certain "designated health services" payable by Medicare to an entity that the physician, or an immediate family member of the physician, has an investment interest in or a compensation arrangement with; and (2) prohibits the entity from submitting claims with Medicare (or fee-for-service Medicaid programs) for those referred services, unless the arrangement satisfies an exception that is described in the Act or the Final Regulations.

The government is not required to prove an unlawful intent—only that the arrangement exists and that it does not satisfy at least one exception included in the statute or regulations.

Exceptions to the Stark Law

The statute provides for three general categories of exceptions to this prohibition. The first category of exceptions applies to both ownership/investment interests and compensation arrangements, the second category applies only to ownership/investment interests, and the third category applies only to compensation arrangements.

However, the complexity of the health care system has made it very difficult for CMS to promulgate exceptions that will provide the "bright line" clarity envisioned by Congressman Stark when he proposed that law. As a result, CMS has issued, and will continue to issue, regulations that will define key terms, alter the interpretation of the Stark law and add new exceptions.

Sanctions

The Stark law is a strict liability statute and, as stated above, intent is irrelevant. Medicare has the right to deny payment for any claim submitted by a provider for any "Designated Health Services" provided pursuant to a referral that does not comply with one of the exceptions to the Stark law. It is also possible for the government to assess civil money penalties and exclusions due to a violation of the Stark law.

In addition, a violation of the Stark law may be found to violate the federal False Claims Act ("FCA"). Penalties for violation of the FCA include three times the amount of the claim, plus a civil penalty of not less than $5,500 or more than $11,000 per claim. Private parties may bring an FCA action under the so-called "qui tam" rules that permit the private party to share in the amount recovered.

Designated Health Services

The "Designated Health Services" ("DHS") covered by the Stark Law include clinical laboratory; physical therapy; occupational therapy; radiology or other diagnostic services; durable medical equipment; parenteral and enteral nutrients, equipment, and supplies; prosthetics, orthotics, and prosthetic devices; home health; outpatient prescription drugs; and inpatient and outpatient hospital services. The list of DHS is updated annually and may be found at http://www.cms.hhs.gov/PhysicianSelfReferrals/11Listofcodes.asp#TopofPage.

Financial Relationship

"Financial relationship" is defined as any direct or indirect *ownership* or *investment* interest in a DHS entity to which the physician refers or any *compensation arrangement* with a DHS entity involving either the physician or an immediate family member of the physician.

Ownership and investment interests include equity, debt, or other interests. They also include interests in the DHS entity that holds an ownership or investment interest in the entity providing the service.

Compensation arrangements include any arrangement involving any remuneration between a physician (or immediate family member) and a DHS entity. Remuneration may be direct or indirect, overt or covert, paid in cash or in kind. Thus, such things as forgiveness of debt, provision of services or space at other than market value, or an indirect return on investment would be considered to be remuneration in the same way as an outright payment of cash.

The Stark regulations define the term "financial relationship" to include "direct or indirect" compensation arrangements or ownership interests. A "direct" financial relationship exists where remuneration flows directly from the entity providing designated health services to the physician without any intervening entity or person. An "indirect" financial relationship exists when remuneration flows through an "unbroken chain" of persons or entities between the DHS entity and the individual physician. Thus, attempting to channel otherwise prohibited financial relationships through a parent-subsidiary corporate arrangement will not avoid the law. Attempts to use intermediate entities to avoid the scope of the Stark law was made even more difficult when CMS added its so-called "Stand in the Shoes" rules under which CMS may impute a direct compensation arrangement to exist notwithstanding the presence of any number of intermediate entities.

Investment Interests

Because of the scope of the Stark law, physician investment in DHS entities to which the physician makes referrals is limited. Since the Stark Law only applies to entities that provide a DHS, it will not apply to physician investments in an entity that does not provide DHS, such as an ambulatory surgical center. There is an exception for investment in DHS entities located in rural areas, and while, as will be discussed below, the exception has been limited by the Health Reform Law, there is an exception that allows certain physicians to have an ownership interest in a hospital in which they practice. There is also an exception that permits physicians to invest in the group practice in which they provide services.

The definition of a DHS entity was expanded on October 1, 2009, to include the entity that performs a DHS as well as the entity that billed for the DHS. This change has greatly expanded the number of entities to which the Stark law applies and in doing so has significantly decreased opportunities for physician investment.

Compensation Arrangements

Compensation arrangements are essentially contractual arrangements between DHS entities and a physician (or immediate family member). The Stark law divides compensation arrangements into two broad categories: (1) employment and (2) independent contractor relationships. The exception that must be satisfied depends on which broad category applies.

Employment

Under the Stark rules, employment relationships are given special status. An employer may attempt to qualify as a physician group if it is an entity that is separate from a hospital or other DHS entity and can be organized and operated in the manner described in 42 C.F.R. §411.352. If a group practice is involved, physician compensation may include in-office ancillary services, incident-to payments and revenues generated by other physicians in the group, to the extent and in the manner permitted by the Stark regulations.

There is a separate employment exception for a DHS entity that either chooses not to form, or does not qualify as, a group practice. This is the exception a hospital must use if it employs a physician directly. This employment exception permits the employer to pay the physician a productivity bonus. However, the bonus is limited to "services personally performed by the physician." As such, that bonus may not include in-office ancillary services, "incident-to" services, or revenue generated by other physicians. This limitation on the productivity bonus is the biggest difference between a physician who is employed pursuant to the employment exception and one who is employed in a group practice.

While it is a good idea to use a written employment agreement, employment is one of the few compensation arrangements where the applicable Stark exceptions do not require a written agreement. However, regardless of whether the employment agreement is written or oral, the employment must be for identifiable services and the amount of remuneration paid to the employee must be consistent with fair market value, commercially reasonable, and not determined in a manner that takes into account (directly or indirectly) the volume or value of referrals by the physician.

Independent Contractor Relationships

The intrinsic flaw with the Stark statute is that it attempts to pigeonhole relationships between physicians and DHS entities. Under the statute, if the arrangement does not fit into a specific pigeonhole, it is prohibited. However, many beneficial relationships do not always fit neatly into the categories included in the statute. While the DHS entity needs to locate at least one "pigeon hole," there are certain requirements that are common to most of the exceptions that apply to non-employed physicians (i.e., Independent Contractors), including: the transaction must be in writing that is signed by both parties, describe the services covered by the agreement, and specify a time frame for the arrangement, which generally (although not always) is at least one year. The compensation specified in the agreement must be prospective in nature, consistent with fair market value, be set in advance and not take into account the volume or value of any referrals generated by the parties, and not violate any other federal or state law, such as the anti-kickback statute.

The Stark exceptions that apply to independent contractors include, but are not limited to: the lease of space or equipment; personal service agreements such as medical director agreements or on-call agreements; isolated transactions, such as the site of a practice, recruitment agreements; retention arrangements in rural areas; compliance training and the donation of electronic medical records.

Medical Staff Specific Exceptions

There are also exceptions to the Stark law that attempt to address the unique relationship between a hospital and the physicians who are appointed to the hospital's medical staff. The non-monetary compensation exception is one such exception and the medical staff incidental benefits exception is another.

Nonmonetary Compensation Exception

This exception permits compensation in the form of items or gifts (but not cash or cash equivalents) that do not exceed the then applicable limit in any calendar year adjusted for inflation. When this exception was adopted, this amount was $300. However, it has been subject to an annual adjustment for inflation. After the inflation adjustment, the 2007 calendar year amount was $329; the 2008 calendar year amount was $338; it was

$355 in calendar years 2009 and 2010; and $359 in calendar year 2011. CMS updates this amount annually and the current annual limit may be found at http://www.cms.hhs.gov/PhysicianSelfReferral/10-CPI-U-Updates.asp.

Even when adjusted for inflation, the annual limit makes this exception of limited utility. Furthermore, in order to satisfy this exception, the hospital must track all such items or gifts, the item or gift must not be determined in any manner that takes into account the volume or value of referrals or business generated by the referring physician, may not be solicited by the physician, and cannot violate the Anti-Kickback Statute.

Additional refinements to this exception include: (1) no more often than once every three years, a physician who has inadvertently received non-monetary compensation of up to 50% in excess of the then applicable limit may repay the excess within the earlier of the same calendar year or 180 days of receipt of the excess, and (2) a DHS entity may provide one medical staff function per year for the entire medical staff without regard to any monetary limit. While the cost of the annual medical staff event is not counted against the then annual limit, any gifts or gratuities provided in connection with that event (including "door prizes") will be subject to the annual limit.

Medical Staff Incidental Benefits Exception

The Stark exceptions also include a "Medical Staff Incidental Benefits" exception. While it is helpful that CMS has recognized that the regulations should include an exception that recognizes a number of traditional relationships between a hospital and the physicians who are appointed to its medical staff, this exception is still relatively narrow and has a number of requirements, including the requirements that the item or services: be offered to all staff members practicing in the same specialty without regard to the volume or value of their referrals to the hospital; be provided only during periods when the medical staff members are making rounds or are engaged in other activities that benefit the hospital or its patients; and, with very limited exceptions, must be used by the medical staff member on the hospital's campus, be reasonably related to the delivery of medical services at the hospital, and not be intended to induce referrals.

Also, the compensation must be of low value. Originally, each item was valued at $25 and has been subject to the same inflation adjustment that is used in the non-monetary compensation exception. In calendar year 2007, this amount was adjusted to $28 per occurrence; it was increased to $29 per occurrence in calendar year 2008; and $30 per occurrence in calendar years 2009, 2010 and 2011. Future updates can be found at the same area of the CMS website as the update for non-monetary compensation.

This is the so-called "free lunch exception." Therefore, assuming that all of the requirements to the exception are met, a hospital may provide free meals, free parking, or any other "on campus" incidental benefit that it normally provides to all members of its medical staff practicing in the same specialty without fear that that benefit will be construed as a prohibited compensation arrangement, as long as the value of each individual benefit (i.e., each meal) is less than the then applicable per item limit (i.e., $28 during calendar year 2007, $29 in 2008, or $30 in 2009, 2010 and 2011) even if the aggregate value of all of the benefits provided to a physician over the course of a calendar year exceeds the then applicable limit for nonmonetary compensation (i.e., $329 for calendar year 2007; $338 in calendar year 2008; $355 in calendar years 2009 and 2010; or $359 in calendar year 2011).

Health Care Reform

The Patient Protection and Affordable Care Act is an omnibus federal law that affects a number of areas and is being phased in over time. The key provisions of the law include mandated coverage for individuals and employers with penalties for non-compliance (the "individual mandate"); minimum coverage requirements for insurers; creation of insurance exchanges; subsidies for individual coverage; and expansion of Medicaid eligibility.

This law also amended the fraud and abuse laws described above in a number of ways, including mandating reporting and repayment of overpayment from Federal Health Care Programs; requiring physicians groups to provide notice to patients before referring the patient for in-office PET, MRI or CT Services; imposing restrictions on the ability of a physician to invest in a hospital; and adding new requirements for tax-exempt hospitals.

The Health Care Reform Law has been subject to a number of legal challenges of one type or another. The Individual Mandate Case has proven to be the most controversial section of this bill. At the time this article is being written, there exists a split in the Federal Circuit Courts as to the constitutionality of the law and/or certain of its sections, most particularly, the Individual Mandate. As a result, the Supreme Court will have the last say on whether the Health Reform Law will be found to be a constitutional exercise of congressional authority.

Chapter 9

Health Informatics for the Physician Executive

by David Masuda, MD, MS

"Few of us doubt...that we are witness to and are part of...an intellectual revolution...with double fault lines crossing from information technology and health...."[1]

Introduction

The physician new to the executive suite not uncommonly experiences symptoms of vertigo and dizziness—symptoms consistent with a common ailment in medical professionals who take on the boundary-spanning physician executive role. It is the distinctly unpleasant feeling of one's head spinning. Enterprise leadership can be a new and unfamiliar experience for most physicians and it not surprising that entrants feel overwhelmed and frustrated. These emotions are brought on not only by the breadth of the new knowledge and skills required in the role, but also by the pace of change in the health care environment. The medical profession has endured an unsettling evolution in how medicine is practiced, measured, regulated, perceived, valued, and reimbursed. Almost certainly this trend will continue, if not accelerate. The pace of change in health care has not been an easy one for physicians or managers to accept or adapt to, yet as Chute so clearly observes,[1] it is not only the rapid evolution of medicine with which physicians must contend. The pace of change in informatics, a fundamentally important knowledge domain of the physician executive, may be even more disorienting. As we will discuss in this chapter, the rapid change in informatics will intensify the physician executive's sense of confusion and disorientation. These double fault lines make for shaky ground beneath the physician executive's feet.

The Health Care Environment

Health care in the United States is becoming increasingly unaffordable because of rising costs for employers and consumers and increasingly unattainable for a growing number of citizens who are uninsured or under-insured. A major component of this cost growth is due to high-technology developments across the spectrum of care, especially in pharmaceuticals. Paradoxically, rising costs appear to be uncorrelated with quality of the care. Regardless of the metric used to define quality, we see few generalizable and widely successful instances of meaningful improvement in quality of care, whether it be patient satisfaction, patient outcomes, or care processes. To make matters worse, two Institute of Medicine reports indicate that the underlying problem is far worse than most of us would have guessed.[2,3] These reports have been deemed a wake-up call to the U.S. health care system (and hence to health care's leadership), making explicit the inherent issue of preventable medical error. One response, evidence-based medicine (EBM), has risen as a driving force in medical training and practice. Yet despite clear evidence that EBM can improve outcomes, adoption remains slow and spotty. All of these factors have led to a response from our patients. Consumer empowerment in health care suggests a fundamental and dramatic change in the nature of the doctor-patient relationship and of the health care system in general. In short, the concepts of cost, quality, accountability, and choice summarize a health care environment for which the metaphor of a train running off the tracks is no longer used only in jest. Clearly a career's worth of challenges are in place for the physician executive.

The Information Technology Environment

More than 30 years ago, Gordon Moore of Intel observed a somewhat surprising feature in the design of silicon-based computer chips, an observation that has since become know as Moore's Law.[4] Moore noted that, in effect, the computing power available to us doubles roughly every 18 months as the price of that computing power is held constant. We live in a world in which exponential change in information technology capability and reach is the norm. Moreover, it seems very likely this rapid pace of computing power growth will continue well into the next decade. There is more raw computing power in the digital greeting card that plays a rendition of "Happy Birthday" than existed on the planet 45 years ago. Our ability to make digital every aspect of what we do is unprecedented, and often unfathomable.

However, this description of computing evolution is incomplete. One of the first lessons an informaticist learns is the general rule that "informatics ≠ computers." While computers are without doubt fundamental to informatics, the change in the information technology environment is due to more than computing alone. In his 1996 book, *The Digital Economy*, Don Tapscott described a convergence of other factors as core to understanding the set of forces in this environment.[5] The three factors Tapscott described are computing, communication, and content. As we've noted, exponential change in computing means faster and cheaper computers on the desktop and across the enterprise year to year. Even more important, it means that what we consider to be a "computer" is changing. Computer chips are becoming ubiquitous, making all manner of devices "intelligent." A quick survey of your hospital or office will almost certainly reveal not only a "computer" on your desk, but as well, dozens of computing devices all around you.

What gives these myriad computing devices true significance is the second of Tapscott's forces, exponential change in communication. The exemplar in communication is the Internet, more specifically the World Wide Web. The Web has changed nearly every aspect of our lives and work. The Internet and the Web enable every computer and every computing device to talk to each other—to share data and information literally anywhere at the speed of light. Ubiquitous computing interconnected by communication channels of global reach results in ubiquitous information. With ubiquitous information, Tapscott considers the third force—exponential change in content. While perhaps less intuitive than computing and communication, rapid development in content may be the most significant factor for the physician executive to consider. Content, in Tapscott's model, refers to anything that can be digitized. Data, information, and knowledge in medicine and health care increasingly can be captured, stored, retrieved, and reused in digital forms.

"Double Fault Lines Crossing"

Health care leaders no longer have the luxury of adopting a laissez-faire approach to strategic planning in information technology. As the pace of change accelerates, health care enterprises, faced with increasing uncertainty, are making concerted efforts at planning for multiple possible future states. While a clear vision of the future of our organizations may be dizzy and confused, one thing is clear—neither of these evolutions is stoppable. It is not within the range of options for the physician executive to disregard or diminish the importance of these changes. It may well be that what is needed is a new way to look at this world.

The Physician Executive World View of Informatics

It seems that there are as many informatics definitions as there are informatics practitioners. The confusion over definitions is a vexing obstacle in that an increasingly broad spectrum of people in health care claim to "do informatics." We are seeing turf wars develop over who is best trained and best skilled to be the recognized resource for informatics. From the perspective of the physician executive, the argument is moot—important work remains to be done. Suffice it to say that the issue may well be less "what is informatics?" and more "who are the people involved, and what do they care about?"

In the view of the traditionalist, the informaticist is best defined as one who sees informatics as a scientific discipline in which the primary goal is furthering the body of knowledge in the domain. Edward Shortliffe has defined it thusly: "Medical Informatics is the rapidly developing scientific field that deals with the storage, retrieval, and optimal use of biomedical information, data, and knowledge for problem solving and decision making."[6] Key to this definition is the concept of informatics' being an academic activity more than an application area. As a field of scientific inquiry, informatics borrows from a number of other scientific disciplines, including computer science, mathematics, engineering, information science, the cognitive sciences, and the management sciences, among others. If we consider informatics to be a more theoretically based pursuit, the more direct application of computing and communications technology in health care contexts might better be termed health care information technology (IT). In practice these two terms are used interchangeably. Of perhaps more practical value to the physician executive is consideration of informatics as it applies to the people in health care who use its tools. Covvey has proposed a helpful categorization. "Health Informaticians (HIs) are professionals that develop and/or deploy systems and methods based on information and communications technologies in support of health care, research, health system administration, and teaching. HIs require a well-developed knowledge base that encompasses the health system, computer science, and health information systems-related topics, as well as a set of intellectual and procedural skills, and preparatory experiences.... We have proceeded with three distinct groups of professionals in mind. There are the Applied Health Informatics (AHI) professionals who are the *solution deployers;* the Research and Development Health Informatics (RDHI) professionals who are the researchers and teachers who *create new capabilities and produce new professionals;* and the Clinicians with Health Informatics (CHI) competence who are the users of the systems in patient care, research, and teaching."[7] In the world view of the physician executive, the applied health informaticians and the clinicians with health informatics competencies are the most significant. To effectively develop and deploy IT, physician executives should be comfortable in both the first and second roles.

In the next section of this chapter we will discuss the nuts and bolts of technology, the range of IT applications important in health care, and the leadership and management implications of these technologies.

Technology

CPUs, optical drives, MIPS, recursive algorithms, object-oriented data-bases, network topologies. The medical student has to learn a lot of new words in the first year of medical school. It is conceivable that the computer and communication technologies pose an equally steep language learning curve. A small number of physicians and physician executives are conversant in both medical and technical language, but the majority of us are not fluent on the technical side. This does not mean that we must become knowledgeable in IT terminology to the same level as we are in medical terminology. When it comes to management of health care information technologies—computer hardware, computer software, database management systems, and communications networks—the physician executive should strive for a *basic* understanding of the language and, more important, the concepts of the technologies so that he or she is able to have meaningful dialog with the technology experts. The successful physician executive must also understand the limits of his or her technology knowledge and know where to go for help once outside that range. Intimidation by technical jargon is not uncommon. Physician executives have often been described as "boundary spanners"—leaders who are able to bridge the cultural and knowledge gap between the clinical world and the administrative world. The physician executive must also be able to span *both* the clinical-information technology gap *and* the administrative-information technology gap.

Health Informatics Applications

As noted above, there is virtually no aspect of medicine or health care in which information technology is not involved. Some areas are more intimately involved than others, but all areas will eventually be integrated with information technology. The goal here is to develop a categorization of these applications such that the physician executive has a better understanding of the reach of IT into all aspects of health care clinical and management arenas. In the following pages one such categorization is presented, following on the work of Austin, who defines four categories of information systems important in health care today—clinical applications, management applications, e-health applications, and decision support applications.[8] These are not fully separate and distinct categories, nor is this the only model for categorization, but it is a useful model for our purposes. It is important to note that, depending on the specific type of health care organization within which you work, the set of applications used, or needed, may vary.

Clinical Applications

Clinical information systems have a primary objective of supporting patient care. Clinical systems include those that are clinician-specific, care location-specific, and technology-specific. Among the oldest clinical applications are those that support individual clinical departments or clinical services in hospitals. Most notable of these are radiology, laboratory, and pharmacy systems. These clinical service applications have been around for decades and continue to evolve in terms of complexity and capability. Historically speaking, each of them has evolved relatively independently, both in terms of the computer technology utilized (minicomputers moving to microcomputers and networked PCs) and in terms of the functions performed (initially only patient tracking and now virtually all patient and staff functions in a department). For example, pharmacy information systems make extensive use of robotics for drug distribution, and radiology information systems are designed around PACs (picture archiving and communications systems) that capture all of a patient's imaging information in digital form. As laboratory, pharmacy, and radiology systems have successfully improved information capture and flow, other clinical departments have begun to develop and utilize information technology applications that answer the unique needs of their departments. The emergency department, the operating room, anesthesia, critical care, labor and delivery, and others are now able to build or buy dedicated systems.

Nursing information systems are an example of clinician-specific systems. These tools provide for patient care planning, critical care monitoring, and general nursing staffing management. In terms of care location-specific systems, ambulatory care information systems have grown in significance. Typified by the systems marketed to physician practices, these tools provide for patient scheduling and appointment functions, billing and financial functions, contract management, materials management, quality management, and clinical functions through an electronic medical record (EMR). Other examples of care location-specific systems are long-term care information systems and home-health information systems.

The most significant clinical application in health care today—one that will demand a significant proportion of the IT time and effort of the physician executive—is the EMR, including its two tightly integrated components, computerized provider order entry (CPOE) and clinical decision support systems (CDSS). Collectively, these applications represent the bulk of hospital and integrated delivery system IT investments, and this will likely remain the case for many years to come. A detailed discussion of EMR/CPOE/CDSS is not possible here. Suffice it to say the reader should strongly consider that this may well be the first IT area to explore further after completing this book. For our purposes, one should consider the EMR as a set of functions that, at one core level, revolve by design around the work of the physician. These tools are designed to support, extend, and enhance what the physician does. By definition then, these tools also change what it is the physician does. This is not a trivial change—human beings react to change in a number of ways, and these reactions often may be counter to organizational goals, to improved patient care, and to the expectations of the physician executive. Because the EMR and CPOE will commonly be a responsibility of many physician executives, it behooves them to be well versed in the change management skills necessary to increase the likelihood of successful adoption.

Management Applications

The clinical information systems described in the last section are a relatively new development in health care when compared to the applications in management information systems. Austin provides a helpful categorization here as well.[8] Perhaps the oldest application in health care is financial information systems, the backbone of health care organizations. These tools support the general operation of the organization and include tools for general and patient accounting, payroll, and management of contracts and investments. Financial systems also allow for management decision making by creating financial reports and forecasts and investment analysis. Another management application area is human resources information systems, with functions that include maintaining employee records; analyzing labor and labor costs; tracking personnel issues, such as absenteeism and turnover; tracking of employee skills and certifications; and monitoring productivity, quality control, and compensation/benefit packages. Resource utilization and scheduling applications monitor occupancy rates, clinical department activity and utilization, and patient and staff scheduling. Materials management applications encompass computerized purchasing using electronic data interchange (EDI), inventory control, and computerized menu planning and food service management. Facilities and project management applications allow for preventive maintenance, construction and remodeling project management and control, and energy conservation. Finally, office automation applications include word processing, document management, electronic mail, teleconferencing, project management, meeting scheduling, and calendar maintenance.

Extending outside of the typical set of hospital-based management information systems are those important to other types of health care organizations. Managed care information systems share much of the functionality of hospital systems but, because managed care systems have a number of significantly different information needs, have additional functionality, such as information on plan benefits and limits; plan membership; claims submission, processing, and adjudication; procedure and specialist visit authorization; and approved provider lists. Finally, integrated delivery systems (IDS) applications (also known as enterprise systems) are increasingly important as the separation between health care organizations becomes less and less distinct. All of the functions described above are important in IDSs. In fact, one of the bigger challenges for IDSs is to be able to effectively link existing systems in all of these areas to other similar systems across the IDS.

e-Health Applications

While applications in the clinical and management domains closely reflect the organizational work of these two primary components of health care, applications in e-health are defined instead by an information technology—specifically, the information technology of the Internet and the World Wide Web. These communications technologies have created an unprecedented opportunity for fundamental transformation in the processes and outcomes of health care.

Finding a definition of the term "e-health" is challenging. It generally indicates the application of Internet and Web communications tools and standards to electronic transactions and information exchange across a wide variety of interactions between people in health care. In this sense, it is perhaps fair to claim that all health is e-health. Eysenbach has nicely captured this transformative potential in writing that e-health "characterizes not only technical development, but also a state-of-mind, a way of thinking, an attitude, and a commitment for networked global thinking, to improve health care locally, regionally, and worldwide by using information and communication technology."[9]

Austin describes four main types of application areas in e-health.[8] These include *e-business* applications in which organizations use the Internet and the Web to streamline procurement and claims processing and to sell goods and services to patients and customers (such as Web-based pharmacies). *Marketing and consumer information* applications include tools that enable Web-based advertising through development and distribution of health care-related information for patients and customers. Hospital websites fall into this category. E-health applications in the *organizational management and communications* category include enterprise intranets used to offer employees easier access to organizational information and to education and training programs. Outside the organization, these systems can be used to recruit new employees. Finally, *clinical and customer service* applications, perhaps the most potentially transformative concept, provide patients direct electronic access to their personal medical records via the Web and to their personal providers via e-mail and secure Web messaging.

Decision Support Applications (DSS)

Arguably the least visible set of applications, yet the one most germane to the activities of physician executives, is the set of applications that provide decision support. Here we are not considering decision support in the form of smart CPOE systems that provide alerts and reminders to physicians as they enter orders for their patients. We are talking about the systems that executives use to better inform managerial decision-making. Austin borrows a categorization system for managerial decision support from Alter, one that defines DSS in terms of[10]:

- Systems in which users retrieve isolated data items
- Systems used as mechanisms for ad hoc analysis of data files
- Systems that provide pre-specified aggregations of data in the form of standard reports
- Systems that assist in estimating the consequence of proposed decisions
- Systems that propose decisions to management
- Systems that make decisions according to predetermined decision algorithms

In isolated data retrieval systems, various databases can be queried for data and information, such as a list of materials vendors or physician contracts. Ad hoc analysis systems are typified by a general statistical package used to quantify data sets. Applications that report pre-specified aggregated data are well known to physician executives and could include reports on drug utilization, admissions, and LOS by physician. Consequence estimation tools allow decision-makers to model "what-if" questions, such as what would be the budgetary and revenue implications of purchasing a new imaging device such as MRI. If such a system is also capable of optimizing these "what-if" queries to suggest the most cost-effective decision, one has a tool that proposes decisions to management. Finally, systems that can make decisions independently are considered "expert systems" and are increasingly playing a significant role in managerial work. Examples of these systems are ICD coders that can assign optimal billing codes on the basis of answers to simple questions about the diagnosis and systems that attempt to detect billing fraud on the basis of subtle differences in how providers bill for services.

Information Technology Management and Leadership

As with each core element of the health care enterprise, information systems require clear and thoughtful strategic planning as well as proactive, watchful, and measured management. While we do have reasonable experience with the latter, the former is a more recent development in health care organizations. In the past, enterprise senior leadership and governance rarely paid much attention to the specifics of IT, generally considering the purpose of IT to be a set of tools primarily to support internal communications and a few key internal operations process. It was common for developments to be uncoordinated, with decisions on standards and systems made at department levels, with no clear planning of how, or even whether, to integrate separate systems. This led to systems that supported quite well the often unique information and communication needs of individual departments but that were unable to satisfy the needs of the larger organization. The current health care environment makes this approach untenable. Hospitals and IDSs have come to understand that the old model of decision-making will prevent them from remaining competitive in the market, and hence they have elevated IT planning to the level of fundamental enterprise strategy. They have also elevated the leader within the IT department from the role of data processing manager to Chief Information Officer. As noted earlier, IT frequently represents the largest percentage of organizational capital budgets, and it is critical to spend these scarce resources wisely.

Austin has described a concise overview of the purposes and process of IT strategic planning that we will summarize here.[8] In terms of definitions, Austin states that IT strategic planning is "The process of identifying and assigning priorities to the applications of information technology that will assist the organization in executing its business plans and achieving its strategic goals and objectives." At least four main objectives are to be achieved in creating such plans. First, a good plan makes explicit the *alignment of the IT plan with organization goals and objectives.* Although this seems inherently obvious, in practice it has been common for IT plans to be designed mostly to support day-to-day operations and not the longer term goals of the organization. Hence, there is little effort to understand how IT can materially aid the organization in reaching its goals. Second, the IT plan must distinctly *define the information requirements and priorities* of the enterprise. In the past, the separate silos of IT in health care organizations tended to collect redundant data with no clear understanding of how to share these data. This is both inefficient and ineffective. Because IT is expensive, organizations must actively define what data information is of most value across the enterprise and create clear plans as to how to acquire, store, and reuse these data and information. Third, it must make explicit the definitions of *the IT infrastructure.* Hardware and software come in a broad range of flavors. To achieve optimal integration of computing and communications tools across the enterprise requires planners to choose system components that will best support organizational functions and to mandate their adoption. Fourth, the plan should make explicit *budgeting and resource allocation.* Because most health care organizations will spend considerable sums acquiring and operating IT in the coming years, planning how to pay for it is paramount.

Although the process of IT strategic planning is not significantly dissimilar to strategic planning in general, a few aspects specific to IT are worth mentioning. A central goal will be for organizations to overcome their significant sins of the past in terms of failure to design integrated information systems. While this may require individual departments to employ systems that are not departmentally optimal, the greater gain for the organization through tighter integration is worth the trade off. In the past, health care organizations had to answer the question of build or buy. Currently the trend is away from custom-designed, in-house development of systems. Because of the complexity of systems integration, it is becoming increasingly unfeasible for health care organizations to develop these systems themselves. Finally, as noted previously, an organization goes through significant change in organization process and culture as integrated information systems are deployed enterprise-wide. These forces make the significance of *end-users and change management* a critically important and yet sadly overlooked aspect of careful planning. Recent history is littered with expensive IT failures, not due to poorly designed technology but instead due to poorly designed change management and failure to recognize the importance of involving end users in the process from the very start.

The Difficult Issues

The discussion to this point might suggest that the inevitable integration of IT into health care will be relative straightforward and relatively pain-free. Nothing could be further from the truth. There are at least three meta-level issues that physician executives must consider as they come to better understand the transformation that IT is bringing to health care. First, to garner optimal benefits from IT, we must develop an understanding of the significance of *industry standards.* Human beings have a marvelous ability to understand each other despite our relatively loose and unstructured forms of communication. Two physicians discussing a patient with "stabbing chest pain" will almost certainly agree a myocardial event is taking place. A computer has no way of knowing if this patient is having a heart attack or if the pain is coming from a knife sticking into the chest wall. For information systems to work well, all stakeholders in health care need to agree on how to develop standardized language and terminologies such that the entire range of health care data and information can be effectively and accurately captured. This is no small feat. Many groups have been working for years to achieve a set of such standards, yet significant work remains. Second, the use of information technology in health care brings with it fundamental questions regarding *information security, privacy, and confidentiality.* These issues existed well before we began keeping patient data in computers, but they take on new significance when computers allow us to make limitless copies of that information and send it virtually anywhere via the Internet. As with many issues in informatics, there is no one right answer in dealing with information security and the expectation of confidentiality. There is always a trade off. We have the ability to make a patient's health care information extremely secure, but the cost is that the information will not be easily accessible by legitimate providers for legitimate uses. Conversely, making information widely available at all the possible points of care would very likely allow optimal care decisions but would increase the risk of less than complete security. It is not yet clear how society will come to weigh the trade-offs of confidentiality versus convenience. Third, e-health carries with it the potential for inequality of access to care—the so-called *digital divide*. There are populations who either cannot or will not use information to access various components of the health care system. If the Internet continues to grow as a communications channel for both administrative and clinical transactions, it is possible that continued growth of e-health applications may enable the creation of one more obstacle to care delivery for several segments of the population.

Conclusions

Physician executives in virtually any organization will increasingly find that informatics and information technology play significant and often mission-critical roles in those organizations. These leaders will need a breadth of knowledge about the various applications available and an ability to learn in depth about applications most meaningful to their organizations and environments. In this chapter we have delineated the breadth, and hinted at the significance. Individual physician executives should use this road map to plan their further education in informatics.

The road is not an easy one compared to other skill sets and knowledge domains the physician executive masters. Take capital finance, for example. While it is not at all a trivial matter to make optimal managerial decisions in capital finance, the basics of the subject are relatively standardized, commonly accepted, and stable. Informatics, on the other hand, suffers from ambiguity in both areas. Decision-making is difficult and the underlying knowledge base is spotty at best and continues to change regularly. To conclude this chapter, we'll suggest some rules of thumb that, more often than not, will guide physician leaders to not make grand errors.

The health care futurist Jeffrey Bauer often notes the need for physician executives to develop new world views.[11] Within the domain of informatics, a "technorealistic" world view is critically important. It is exceedingly easy to believe that IT solutions are the first to be considered in an organization. It is equally easy to misspend millions and tens of millions of dollars on such ill-considered IT. And when large health care organizations are spending upwards of 40% of their capital budgets acquiring new IT, this is not a small risk. These failed strategies are not infrequently due to unexplored world views on the part of key decision makers. In this brief chapter we can only provide a cursory overview of the field of informatics. You can't know it all from reading this chapter, or from reading a dozen tomes. The most we can accomplish in this introduction is to give you an outline of the core issues in the field, and to suggest to you an alternative way of thinking—a general framework of guidelines for considering the issues. Borrowing a concept from artificial intelligence in computer science, we'll suggest a set of heuristics, or rules of thumb. In a job where both worlds are changing very fast, this may be the best advice possible.

Six Informatics Heuristics for Physician Executives

1. There is no place to hide.

If one agrees that Tapscott's Convergence model does fit,[5] health care has always been and will increasingly be an information-intensive industry. Whether we consider the financial, administrative, or clinical information aspects, computing and communication technology will become increasingly more significant and more fundamental as process is first automated and then transformed. Even the processes in health care that ostensibly seem immune to IT will be unlikely to remain that way entirely. The deft hand of the surgeon, it has been said, will never be replaced by a computer. Granted, human presence in the OR is a process that will not change any time soon. Yet that human presence may not be quite so "present" as we generally think. In 2002 a patient in France underwent a successful and uncomplicated cholecystectomy performed by a robot controlled by a surgeon 1,000 miles away. In a very real sense, the technology of the scalpel was enhanced by the addition of a very complicated piece of information technology. And speaking of the scalpel, there is research under way to supply the surgeon with an electronic version of that tool. The haptic scalpel will employ computer-controlled microsensors that can detect extremely subtle differences in tissue density and resistance— differences so subtle they are far below the threshold of sensation in the surgeon's fingertips. Such a scalpel blade, when slowly immersed into a beaker containing oil and water is able to sense when the scalpel tip moves through the interface of the oil above and water below. Such an IT-enabled scalpel may reduce the incidence of inadvertent transection of the common duct, making this a surgical complication of historic interest only. In short, there are no facets of health care organizations in which informatics will not have implications.

2. And yet there is no magic bullet.

If our first heuristic suggests a ubiquity of IT, this should not be construed as suggesting that IT solutions always brings effective solutions or desirable organizational change. In fact, recent history in health care informatics suggests the reverse is often true. Clinical information systems have been deployed in hospitals across the country, and there have been significant successes as measured by improvements in financial, care quality, or patient satisfaction metrics. Yet this experience is far from the norm. A significant number of IT investments do not deliver measurable benefit, and, even more troublesome, instance after instance of IT efforts fail grandly. Western society has an unflagging belief in technology. We look to technology to increase productivity, cure our ills, enrich our assets, and generally improve our lives. This world view is equally pervasive in health care. Physician executives must learn to acknowledge our tendency toward a tunnel vision faith in IT as the first and best solution to our biggest problems. Marshall Ruffin stated that "There is no subject matter more important for physician executives to grasp than medical informatics, because the single largest investment by healthcare organizations in the next 10 years will be in medical informatics technologies…" More than a decade later this statement remains entirely true, yet it is incomplete. For physician executives to make these exceedingly large investments wisely, they must be able to acknowledge our deferential attraction to IT as a panacea, and look clearly and evenly at IT as one of many possible solutions to fundamental problems. In other words, to ask both, "How much should we invest in this IT solution?" and "Should we invest in it at all?"[12]

3. Things are not always what they seem.

Business leader Dee Hock formulated what he has called the Sheep's Law of the Universe: "Everything has both intended and unintended consequences. The intended consequences may or may not happen; the unintended consequences always do."[13] When Alexander Graham Bell invented and commercialized the telephone, his world view was that this information technology would be used primarily as a device for information delivery, with the delivery being a one-way process from the information holder to the listener. It never occurred to him that people might want to use the telephone as a tool to chat with their neighbor down the street or a relative in the next state. Introducing IT into health care organizations can have equally unpredictable consequences. Consider the potential effect of the Internet on the doctor-patient relationship. Health care organizations are designing and deploying patient-centric Web sites and patient-provider e-mail to attract new patients and retain current patients. Intended consequences of these Internet IT strategies are that e-mail can replace the telephone call to report lab results and deliver follow-up instructions, potentially alleviating the vexing problem of telephone tag. A patient-centric Web site can enable patients to access more information about the health care organization and their medical problems. The Internet and e-mail have had unintended consequences as well. Patients are able to and choose to bypass their physicians and health care organizations altogether for a number of their health care needs. The Web has provided patients with unprecedented access to medical knowledge. E-mail has allowed for the creation of virtual support groups across the globe, often giving patients precisely what they do not feel they get from their health care organizations—information the patient can understand, time, and compassion.

4. Big I, little t.

Technology is exciting. Information technology can be downright seductive. As a symbol of physician-hood, it would not be entirely surprising to see the PDA become an equal to the stethoscope. The physician who does not use the Web is a relative rarity. At the organizational level, the infiltration of information technology is similarly rapid. Computers are finding their way to the bedside and the exam room. The subject is a common one for the op-ed cartoonist—a sure sign that a social trend has taken hold. A recent cartoon depicted a white-coated physician and a horn-rimmed computer technician standing next to a complex blinking and beeping computing device, both with looks of admiration. The caption reads, "I don't know what you can use it for, Doc, but it sure is high-tech!" When considering information technology, we often fail to realize that the reason we need these tools is to capture, store, and deliver better information so that we can make better and more timely administrative and clinical decisions. We may jump prematurely to the question, "Which vendor's EMR should we buy?" without first exploring the question, "What are the information needs our providers face in their efforts to deliver better care?" When we consider IT, think Big I, little t.

5. The real problem is the meatware.

Despite all of the frustrations we encounter when implementing IT in hospitals and clinics, today's hardware, software, and networks are truly amazing technology. In fact, when it comes to purely technical problems with technology, relatively few problems cannot be solved as long as we are willing to pay for a bit more technology. And this is the exactly the rub. When IT projects go awry, managers, perhaps too quickly, turn to technology-based solutions to the IT project problem. Usually the underlying obstacle or challenge has little to do with the technology per se. The problem is the "meatware"—the people who must use the technology. Octo Barnett, a founding father of medical informatics, has claimed that perhaps 80 percent of informatics failures are due to people and organization issues, not the technology itself.[14] Fortunately, this is good news. While programmers, analysts, and developers in the IT department tend to be both less skilled and disinterested in the people and organizational issues involved in informatics failures, these issues are typically well within the knowledge and skill set of the physician executive. It follows that a primary opportunity for the physician executive is to remind the IT project team that equal consideration is due to both the technical and the human challenges.

6. Paving the cow path.

Old world views are hard to shake. When decision-makers in health care envision how to best implement IT tools to improve the process of work in their organizations, it is common to envision work "the way we currently do it." Subsequently, the technology we employ is designed to make what we currently do more efficient—to automate current process and practice. In taking this perspective, we may fail to consider whether current process and practice are themselves fundamentally problematic. Adding IT to any such suboptimal organizational process or practice workflow can substantially limit the benefit of IT. A paved cow path is still a cow path. This is not to say that automation is without benefit. It is simply to say that the potential of IT is realized when we consider it as a path to organizational transformation. A key concept for the physician executive is to consider the future organization to be one that may look entirely different from the current organization if IT is perceived as an agent of change.

References

1. Chute, C. "The Copernican Era of Health Care Terminology: A Re-Centering of Health Information Systems." *Proceedings of the AMIA Symposium,* 1988.

2. Kohn, L., and others, Editors. *To Err Is Human.* Washington, D.C.: National Academy Press, 2000.

3. Institute of Medicine. *Crossing the Quality Chasm.* Washington, D.C.: National Academy Press, 2001.

4. Moore, G. "Cramming More Components onto Integrated Circuits." *Electronics* 38(8), April 19, 1965.

5. Tapscott, D. *The Digital Economy: Promise and Peril in the Age of Networked Intelligence.* New York, N.Y.: McGraw-Hill, 1997.

6. Shortliffe, E. *Medical Informatics: Computer Applications in Health Care and Biomedicine.* New York, N.Y.: Springer Verlag, 2000.

7. Covvey, H. *Computers in the Practice of Medicine.* Reading, Mass.: Addison-Wesley Publishing, 1980.

8. Austin, C., and others. *Information Systems for Healthcare Management,* 6th Edition. Chicago, Ill.: Health Administration Press, 2003.

9. Eysenbach, G. "What Is E-Health?" *Journal of Medicine Internet Research* 3(2):E20, April-June 2001.

10. Alter, S. *Information Systems: Foundation of E-Business.* Englewood, N.J.: Prentice Hall, 2002.

11. Bauer, J. *Not What the Doctor Ordered: Reinventing Medical Care in America.* Chicago, Ill.: Probus Publishing, 1994.

12. Ruffin, M. "Medical Informatics and the Physician Executive." *New Leadership in Health Care Management: The Physician Executive.* Tampa, Fla.: American College of Physician Executives, 1994, pp. 201-9.

13. Hock, D. *Birth of the Chaordic Age.* San Francisco, Calif.: Berrett-Koehler Publishing, 2000

14. Barnett, O. "Computers in Medicine." *JAMA* 263(19):2631-3, May 16, 1990.

David Masuda MD, MS, currently holds a joint appointment at the University of Washington as lecturer in the Department of Medical Education and the Department of Health Services. He holds an appointment as Senior Lecturer in the Department of Preventive Medicine at the University of Wisconsin-Madison. He is a member of the faculty of the American College of Physician Executives (ACPE), where he has participated in informatics training and curriculum development.

Chapter 10

Fiscal Management of Provider Organizations: Part I

by Hugh W. Long, MBA, PhD, JD
and Mark Covaleski, PhD, CPA

Fiscal or financial management covers a broad spectrum of activities associated with the economics of an organization. Fiscal management encompasses tasks such as writing down in monetary terms a record of the organization's actual historical activity; analyzing that past performance; determining a variety of "costs" for a product or unit of service; raising money for short-term or long-term purposes; designing future performance goals (budgeting); forecasting changes in local or national economic environments and assessing how such changes will affect the organization and how the organization should respond to such changes; and, finally, making resource allocation decisions, both small (how much cash should we have in the bank) and large (should we undertake a $50 million expansion).

The two major organizational fiscal management domains are accounting and finance, each of which covers a wide and diverse range of activities. While "to account" literally means "to keep a record of," accounting encompasses a great deal more than simply keeping records. Similarly, the literal meaning of "to finance" is to gather money for some particular use (e.g., meet a payroll, buy a piece of equipment), but finance involves much more than simply amassing stacks of money.

Much of what accounting and finance address is quite distinct. For example, the information gathering and processing used to generate traditional financial statements (e.g., income statements and balance sheets) has virtually no overlap at all with the information gathering and processing used for asset acquisition analyses. These two distinct fiscal activities, the first a part of accounting, the second a part of finance, are built on quite separate and different sets of concepts and assumptions. As discussed below, using finance cash-flow concepts to define "income" would be as misleading as using financial accounting mechanisms for asset acquisition decisions. Serious errors, indeed irrational outcomes, would result. Hence, identifying the distinct characteristics and uses of each set of tools is a major priority for managers. At the same time, some areas of accounting and finance are closely related, indeed are highly complementary. Much of what managerial accounting addresses requires the same kind of forecasting, modeling, and "what if" analysis that is also central to corporate finance.

This chapter and the next will address these two domains. A combined bibliography for the two domains appears at the end of the next chapter. We begin in this chapter with accounting. In particular, the purposes of this chapter are to:

- Introduce you to some very basic aspects of financial and managerial accounting and what various accounting professionals do.

- Provide you some familiarity with financial accounting information as reflected in company financial statements and the uses of these financial statements.

- Give you some understanding of managerial accounting information as reflected in the company's cost accounting system and the uses of this cost information.

Accounting and Accounting Systems

As suggested above, the field of accounting involves many subspecialties. Internal to health care and other business organizations, one finds financial accounting and managerial and/or cost accounting. Financial accounting has the primary role of keeping records and preparing financial statements; managerial accounting addresses budgeting and control issues (budgeting is really a form of making very short-term resource allocation decisions); and cost accounting identifies costs throughout the organization, allocating those costs to various services or programs (units of output). Other accounting subspecialties include actuaries, who make statistical predictions about the frequency with which certain events (e.g., number of births during a one-year period for a specified population group) may take place; tax accountants, who specialize in working with the income tax code and regulations; and, in the health care industry, accountants, who specialize in the technical aspects of health insurance and payment systems. Accounting firms use certified public accountants (CPAs) to audit the financial statements of client organizations to certify the validity of those statements in accordance with certain rules. CPAs, and often certified management accountants (CMAs), also provide consulting services related to the fiscal management of the organization.

Financial Accounting

The Users of Financial Accounting Information

Financial accounting information is the result of a process of identifying, measuring, recording, and communicating the economic events of an organization (business or nonbusiness) to interested users of the information. This information is summarized and presented in three important financial statements: the balance sheet, the income statement, and the statement of cash flows. Because these statements communicate financial information about an enterprise, accounting is often called "the language of business." An understanding of financial statements provides the users of this information with important insights as to the economic status of the health care organization.

The predominant users of financial accounting information—investors and creditors—have a direct financial interest in evaluating the economic status of the health care organization. Other parties, such as taxing authorities, regulatory agencies, labor unions, customers, and economic planners, may have an indirect financial interest in the economic status of the health care organization and would also be users of financial accounting information. However, our major concern is to understand financial accounting from the eyes of investors and lenders.

Investors typically represent the predominant financial interest in a health care organization. One of the unique features of the health care industry relative to many other industries is that the term "investor" reflects a variety of different forms, depending on the mission of the health care organization. Investors might literally purchase stock in the case of a for-profit health care organization where the shares of stock are sold publicly. However, the term "investors" in the health care industry might also cover situations in which there is no stock, as in classic not-for-profit organizations such as religious-based health care systems, community hospitals, or large not-for-profit private systems. These traditional not-for-profit health care organizations have no explicit investor groups (as reflected by shares of stock), but they can represent their communities at large (whether defined in terms of religious, geographical, or common interests) that have donated and generated wealth for the organizations over the years, thus implicitly representing investor groups. While these implicit investor groups do not receive financial remuneration, such as dividend payments, for their investments, the investing community expects not-for-profit organizations to reciprocate through such paybacks as charity care, support of research, community education, etc.

The critical commonality across these different types of investor groups in the health care industry is that they all have boards of directors.

Whether the health care organization is for-profit or not-for-profit, or issues stock or does not issue stock, the board of directors has a critical fiscal stewardship responsibility—ensuring the economic viability of the health care organization for the broader investors who own the organization. The relationship of investor to organization through financial accounting information becomes crystallized or operationalized in the relationship between the board of directors and the management of the health care organization. Exploiting charitable assets for personal gain can take place in health care organizations if fiscal stewardship by board members is not upheld. Someone has to be watching the store.

Lenders constitute the second broadly defined group that has a direct financial interest in the economic status of the health care organization in the form of the resources that the lending group has provided to the organization. As one of the two dominant sources of financial capital for the health care organization, lenders expect remuneration. Such remuneration is not in the form of a cash dividend, enhancement of economic value of stock (capital appreciation), or a metaphorical dividend such as charity care to the community that the investor group might receive. It is in the form of interest payments received by the lenders from the health care organization. Lenders represent their direct financial interests through the contract of the debt instrument (debt covenants), which often specifies financial results that must be achieved by management and clear consequences for failure to achieve them.

Although these two groups—investors and creditors—are critical users of financial accounting information as a result of their direct financial interests, they do not simply read the financial statements. They can also actively pressure management and the health care organization to achieve desired financial results within these financial statements. This pressure eventually becomes translated into the internal management structure of the health care organization in the form of budgets, pricing strategies, cost cutting strategies, and the like.

Regulation and Standards in Financial Accounting

As a consequence of the Great Depression of the 1930s and the resultant widespread collapse of businesses and the securities market, the federal government intervened and began regulating financial statements and accounting standards. A direct result of this collapse in the financial markets was the creation of the Securities and Exchange Commission (SEC) as an independent regulatory agency. The SEC has the legal power to enforce the form and content of financial statements for companies that wish to sell securities to the public. To do this, the SEC has developed a common set of standards, called generally accepted accounting principles (GAAP), to govern preparation and presentation of financial statements. These principles apply to the area of financial accounting as distinct from other areas of accounting, such as managerial accounting and tax accounting. If a company does not follow GAAP, it will not be allowed to issue securities. The SEC believes that financial statements that follow GAAP provide investors, creditors, and other interested parties with useful information to make informed decisions.

For the most part, the SEC has delegated responsibility for establishing GAAP to a rule-making body called the Financial Accounting Standards Board (FASB). FASB is a private organization whose mission is to establish and improve standards of financial accounting and reporting. Just because FASB has the authority from the SEC and the private resources to study and rule on different financial reporting issues does not guarantee that members of the accounting profession will carry out their work in the manner prescribed by FASB. The American Institute of Certified Public Accountants (AICPA) derives the actual rules and documents (for example, there is an Audit Guide for the Health Care Industry) that public accounting firms and individual CPAs follow when auditing an organization's financial statements. The auditor's report is a letter from the outside auditor giving an opinion on whether or not the firm's financial statements are a fair presentation of the firm's results of operations, cash flows, and financial position in accordance with GAAP. Essentially, these AICPA rulings and audit guides govern the accounting profession and align the work of professional accountants with GAAP. Public accounting firms or individual CPAs who choose not to follow AICPA rulings and documents are subject to strong sanctions by AICPA. In turn, if AICPA rulings and documents stray too far from GAAP, the profession runs the risk of facing the wrath of the SEC.

The Accrual Concept

A critical issue in the financial accounting model pertains to the measurement of the economic event. For example, let us say that an organization provides $700 worth of services in November and does not receive payment until February of the next year. Because the delay crosses over the December 31 fiscal year end, there will be two different accounting results, depending on whether one is using the cash or the accrual basis of accounting.

Under the cash basis of accounting, the organization does not recognize the revenue until the cash is received in February. The argument here is that the critical event is the receipt of cash. The accrual concept states that earned revenue does not necessarily correspond to the receipt of cash. Earned revenue is recognized when a service has been provided and creates a corresponding economic obligation by the purchaser. The asset received in exchange for the services performed may be cash (or some other thing of value), but more often it is accounts receivable. The accrual basis of accounting calls the critical event the provision of service in November. The concern under the accrual accounting method ties back to our discussion of the objectives of financial statements. The argument is that the cash basis of accounting has failed to portray the economic status of the organization. In this case, it can be argued that the cash basis of accounting has understated revenue by $700 in November and overstated it by $700 in February.

So how does the accrual basis propose to remedy this problem. First, the accrual basis will recognize $700 in revenue in November, even though the cash has not yet been received. The asset that will be booked in lieu of cash will be accounts receivable, which, in theory, is almost as good as cash. This recognizes revenue when the service has been provided and matches revenue with the proper period. The slight tradeoff the accrual basis has made is in terms of objectivity; that is, the $700 in accounts receivable may not all eventually translate into cash because of bad debts. Nonetheless, the accounting profession is comfortable enough with the benefits of the tradeoff to recommend accrual basis accounting over cash basis accounting in GAAP. In short, we book (make an entry, in this case debit) $700 to the balance sheet as an asset in the form of accounts receivable and book (credit) $700 to the income statement as revenue in the form of patient services revenue.

Taking this illustration further, when the cash does arrive in February, the accrual basis of accounting can handle this fairly easily in its bookkeeping. Most important is not to double count the revenue. The bookkeeping entries go like this: we book (debit) $700 to the balance sheet as an asset in the form of cash and book (credit) $700 to the balance sheet in the form of a deduction from accounts receivable, thus bringing our accounts receivable balance down to $0. Accounts receivable serves as a bridge (setting it up in November, taking it down in February) that divorces revenue recognition in November from receipt of cash in February. When we receive the cash in February, we do not book revenue again but simply exchange assets—bring in (increase) cash and take down (reduce) accounts receivable.

Let's follow the accrual versus cash basis debate through on the expense side. Let's assume that the organization had payroll obligations of $400 for the last two weeks of December that did not get paid until January. Since this delay crosses over the December 31 fiscal year end, there will again be two different results. The cash basis of accounting does not recognize the expense until the cash is paid—January. The argument here is that the critical event is the payment of cash. The accrual basis of accounting argues that the critical event is the economic obligation related to services provided to the organization by its employees in December. In this case, it can be argued that the cash basis of accounting has understated expenses by $400 in December and overstated these expenses by $400 in January. So how does the accrual basis propose to remedy this problem? First, in December, the accrual basis will recognize a $400 expense even though the cash has not yet been paid. The item that will be booked in lieu of the take down of cash will be a liability—accrued expenses—which, in theory, is a short-term obligation that will need to be paid from cash. This recognizes the expense when the service has been provided and matches expenses to the proper period. We book (debit) $400 to the income statement in the form of salary expense and book (credit) $400 to the balance sheet in the form of accrued expenses.

When the cash does get paid out in January 2000, the accrual basis of accounting can handle the transaction fairly easily. Most important is to not double count the expense. The bookkeeping entries go like this: We book (credit) $400 to the balance sheet as a deduction from an asset (a deduction of cash) and book (debit) $400 to the balance sheet in the form of a removal from the accrued payroll expense liability, thus bringing our accrued expenses balance down to $0. The accrued expenses account serves as a bridge (setting it up in December, taking it down in January) that divorces the expense recognition in December from the receipt of cash in January. When we pay out the cash in January, we do not book payroll expense again but simply make exchanges in the balance sheet—pay out cash (decrease assets) and take down accrued expenses (decrease liabilities).

Appendix A to this Chapter (page 191) presents an introduction to the basic financial accounting statements and their analysis.

Managerial and Cost Accounting

As important as the statements produced by financial accounting systems are, other analyses of the information amassed by the accounting system are even more important for internal managerial purposes. In addition, organizations typically engage in various extensions of financial accounting activity in the form of cost accounting and budgeting. Although cost accounting is sometimes viewed as a subset of managerial accounting, managerial and cost accounting together deal with formulating budgets, analyzing actual fiscal performance in comparison to what was budgeted, projecting the effects of management decisions on future financial accounting statements, identifying actual costs of producing services, calculating "full" costs of services using cost allocation formulas, and dealing with other related issues of cost and payment (e.g., internal transfer pricing, income distribution mechanisms, and maximizing third-party payments). The sections that follow offer a survey of managerial and cost accounting activities.

Cost Concepts

Cost Behavior

Preparation of a budget requires a basic understanding of cost behavior in relation to volume and, as will be discussed later, in terms of responsibility centers. Costs can be expressed as they relate to changes in activities such as occupancy rates, patient visits, patient mix, services provided, etc. Costs described in terms of activity levels (volume) are usually separated in terms of fixed and variable components. A fixed cost is a cost that does not change within the relevant range of alternative levels of activity.* For example, the manager's salary typically will not change with the number of patients. This does not mean it cannot be changed, but it changes as a function of management decisions rather than of activity level. Variable costs, on the other hand, are costs that vary directly with volume. For example, raw food costs will vary with the number of meals served, the costs of pharmacy items can vary with the number of procedures performed, etc. These types of costs are illustrated graphically in figure 1, below.

Figure 1. Total Cost Curves

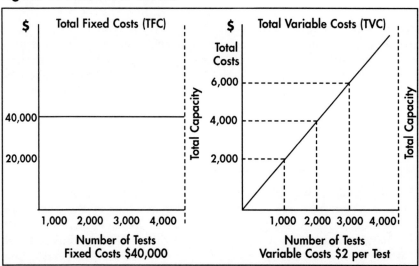

The manager must work with per unit comparisons in addition to the total costs approach displayed in figure 1. Costs are typically expressed on a per unit basis for reimbursement, rate setting, and billing activities. Total costs are a combination of variable and fixed costs; total costs per unit are a combination of variable costs per unit and fixed costs per unit. On a per unit basis, variable costs are the same for each unit of service. For example, if the reagents required for one test are $2.00, they are $4.00 for two tests, $6.00 for three tests, etc. The average or per unit cost remains at $2.00 regardless of volume. This cost relationship can be expressed graphically, as shown in figure 2, below.

In determining total costs per unit, determination of the fixed costs component presents a more difficult challenge, complicated by the large proportion that fixed costs represent of total costs in the health care industry. Because fixed costs per unit are obtained by dividing total fixed costs by the level of activity, the more units provided, the lower the fixed costs per unit. Continuing our test example, suppose the laboratory supervisor is paid $40,000. At a volume of 1,000 tests, this calculates to $40 per test. But fixed costs per unit for 2,000 tests would be $40,000 divided by 2,000, or $20 per test. As most experienced managers have observed, volume is of vital concern for financial well-being because of the heavy fixed cost nature of most health care services. The relationship of per unit fixed costs to volume is illustrated in figure 3, below.

Figure 2. Per Test Variable Cost Curve

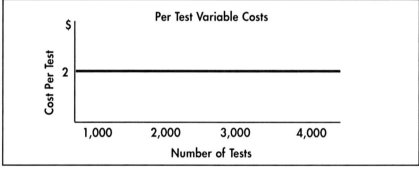

Figure 3. Per Test Fixed Cost

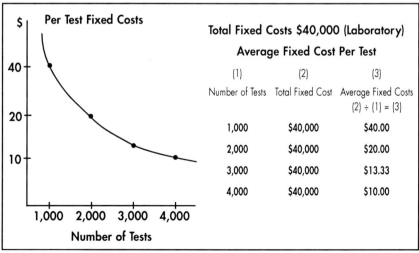

Total Fixed Costs $40,000 (Laboratory)

Average Fixed Cost Per Test

(1) Number of Tests	(2) Total Fixed Cost	(3) Average Fixed Costs (2) ÷ (1) = (3)
1,000	$40,000	$40.00
2,000	$40,000	$20.00
3,000	$40,000	$13.33
4,000	$40,000	$10.00

Figure 4. Average (Full) Cost Determination

(1)	(2)	(3)	(4)
Estimated Number of Tests	Average Variable Cost	Average Fixed Cost $40,000 : Col. (1)	Full Cost Per Test Col. (2) + Col. (3)
1,000	$2	$40.00	$42.00
2,000	2	$20.00	$22.00
3,000	2	$13.33	$15.33
4,000	2	$10.00	$12.00
5,000	2	$ 8.00	$10.00
6,000	2	$ 6.67	$ 8.67
7,000	2	$ 5.71	$ 7.71
8,000	2	$ 5.00	$ 7.00

Appendix B presents a basic algebraic description of the cost/profit/volume method of analyzing cost behavior. It also presents the contribution model and how the outputs of these models can be used as input to decision making.

Average (Full) Cost Determination

Determination of what a test costs is typically based on the average cost of providing the test (total costs divided by volume = average cost, where total costs = total variable costs + total fixed costs). As discussed above, fixed costs per unit will vary as the level of output or volume changes. Therefore, it is impossible to determine per unit costs without first estimating the level of output. Figure 4, above, presents an analysis of the laboratory example discussed above in which capacity is now assumed to be 8,000 tests for the period covered by the analysis.

Computation of full costs per unit is an important element in establishing prices or rates. The computation depends on the planned fixed costs and estimated volume, because the variable costs component is usually not sensitive to changes in the level of output within the relevant range of output. Hence, if one wants to establish a price or rate that covers the costs (total or per test), the price or rate necessarily relies on the underlying fixed costs and volume assumptions.

Related Cost Definitions

Management must be aware of cost classifications in addition to the fixed and variable cost behavior dichotomy. One of the more useful categorizations is direct and indirect costs. Direct costs can be traced directly to the cost objective being measured. For example, the costs of the laboratory test, whether fixed or variable, are direct costs. Conversely, costs that are necessary but are not directly involved with the test are indirect costs. Examples of indirect costs include senior management salaries and the cost of running the business office. These are part of the total costs of providing the test, but they cannot be traced directly to the test (and, in fact, support other outputs in addition to this test). Still, they must be allocated to this test through some mechanism. The distinction between direct and indirect costs is crucial in responsibility accounting and reporting. By separating costs into direct and indirect categories, managers and supervisors can be held accountable for costs they can control. An example of this type of report is illustrated in figure 5, below. In the figure, even though an overall loss is reported, a $270 positive controllable operating margin has been achieved in terms of direct costs over which departmental personnel have control.

Figure 5. Responsibility Center Reporting

Department Activities for the Month	Dollars	Percentage)
Net Revenues	$3,000	100
Controllable Operating Expenses		
Variable Costs	450	15
Contribution Margin	$2,550	85
Controllable Fixed Costs	$2,280	76
Controllable Operating Margin	$270	9
Allocated Costs	1,500	50
Net Operating Margin (Loss)	($1,230)	(41)

Cost Estimating Techniques

Considerable progress has been made in the recent past in using statistical modeling techniques to estimate costs and cost behavior in health care settings. Most of these techniques involve a form of regression analysis in which independent variables such as patient days are used to predict dependent variables such as nursing hours and supply costs on the basis of historical relationships. For example, a relationship between volume of laboratory tests and supervisory hours could be presented on a scatter diagram as shown in figure 6, page 180. The relatively flat nature of the curve indicates that supervisory hours are fixed for the range of tests covered. The slope of the regression line in figure 7, page 180, indicates that technician hours increase with volume of tests, as common sense would suggest. Supervisors are involved with administration and supervision of

Figure 6.

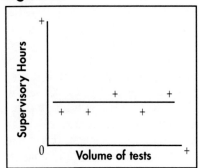

Figure 7.

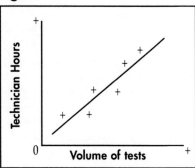

the technicians, while the technicians perform most of the direct work. Statistical techniques can be used to estimate the fixed and the variable portions of the technician hours.

Those who wish to explore these techniques in greater detail are encouraged to review the references for this section at the end of this chapter.

Overhead Costs

Overhead or indirect costs can represent a significant part of the total costs of the health care provider. Costs that cannot be traced directly to the provision of individual patient services typically fall into the overhead area. The salaries of senior management, clerical staff, and accounting staff and general maintenance/housekeeping costs are examples of overhead costs. These costs are difficult to control, because, while they are necessary, they are typically not directly related to the provision of patient services and thus to revenues.

In addition, because there is no direct relationship between revenues and costs, it is difficult to determine the "correct" amount of these costs, i.e., should they be expanded or should they be cut? What should be the size of a business office? How many accountants, clerks, and administrators are needed? What type of equipment do they require? How much space should be allotted to them?

These decisions—and their resultant costs—are not directly related to the number of patient visits, the number of discharges, or the number of procedures performed, but they are an essential part of providing high-quality service to patients. In order to determine the full cost of providing services, it is necessary to devise some method of allocating a "fair" share of overhead costs to each activity being performed.

Allocation Methods

Allocation of overhead costs to the various activities of the organization requires development of an overhead charge per unit of service. Overhead charges are basically "average" shares of total overhead costs that can be applied to the service performed. Total overhead costs can be determined from the budget before the period of operations begins and from the accounting system after the period of operations ends. These total overhead costs are divided by the activity base selected to obtain the overhead charge (total overhead costs divided by volume). Each unit of service thus receives an estimated share of the overhead cost. For example, business office costs could be allocated on the basis of the number of employees in each section. Nursing administration costs could be allocated according to the number of FTE nurses or the level of patient activity. Social service costs could be allocated according to the number of users or the total hours of service received by patients.

Allocation of overhead requires that the health care provider be divided into patient care centers and patient support centers. Patient care centers are departments that provide direct care and for which revenue can be recognized. Support centers are all other activities or cost centers, such as the business office, housekeeping, or marketing.

Summary

In order to determine what a service or an activity costs, it is necessary to define exactly the purpose for which the cost information is being collected. Because of the effect of fixed costs on per unit costs, such cost figures are appropriate only for the volume selected. Statistical techniques are available to assist managers in estimating costs and cost behavior. Overhead costs present special challenges, and choices surrounding overhead allocations can significantly affect calculated per unit total costs.

Pricing Strategies and the Role of Managerial Accounting

An important part of managerial decision making pertains to establishing or accepting a price for health care services. For example, in a fee-for-service environment, health care organizations need to determine whether they should offer discounts for large-volume services to valued payer groups such as large HMOs or business coalitions. In a capitated environment, the health care organization needs to determine the premium amount within which it is willing to risk responsibility for the provision of health care services. And in the case of payers such as Medicare and Medicaid, for which the health care organization is basically a price taker, the organization still needs to know the impact of this de facto decision to sell services to the government. Understanding how to analyze product costs, such as costs by services, costs by DRG classification, or costs by enrollment population, is important for making such pricing decisions. Even when prices are set by overall market supply and demand forces (or by government power) and the health care organization has little or no influence on them, the organization still has to make decisions about the extent and the mix of services offered. An important function of management accounting is to supply cost information that helps support pricing decisions.

Because the financial resources of most health care providers are derived chiefly from revenue received for providing health care services, it is essential that health care managers establish rates or prices that will generate revenues sufficient to meet the organization's total financial requirements. Total financial requirements include the full cost of doing business (operating expenses). However, it is important that revenue provide for the replenishment of existing assets; the costs of assets to expand into new services; and, in the case of a for-profit organization, dividend rewards to investors.

One of the critical underpinnings of past pricing strategies of health care organizations was cross-subsidization, which essentially meant markups (overcharging) on many routine services, such as radiology and ancillary services, and undercharging on other services to support teaching and care for the poor. Such cross-subsidization (also sometimes called "cost-shifting") helped many hospitals to function as full-service institutions. Major purchasers are no longer interested in having cross-subsidies built into their prices to support the provision of health care services to others who are not the purchaser's moral and economic responsibility. Health care organizations that continue to base pricing strategies on extensive cross-subsidization will contribute to two adverse selections:

- Healthier populations will move to providers whose prices reflect real value to purchasers.
- Less healthy populations will move to health care organizations that offer services below value (the difference that has historically been subsidized by other groups or services). This adverse selection will challenge the ability of health care providers to function as full-service institutions.

Today, however, the pricing strategies of health care organizations take place in a much more competitive marketplace. As health care organizations begin to understand the competitive forces driving much of the health care industry, one of their important insights is whether they can influence the price of their health care service/product. If the health care organization is one of many providers in its area and there is little to distinguish its services, economic theory suggests that prices will be set by supply and demand. No health care organization can influence prices significantly by its own decisions. In such a situation, the health care organization may well be a price-taker, because it more or less follows prices set in the market-place. This is probably the case for most health care organizations.

As a general rule, health care organizations that are price-takers need to take the industry price as a given and concentrate on the other two critical variables (cost structure and volume) to affect the fourth variable (profits). This price-taker health care organization should offer as much as it can of its services whose costs are less than the industry price (even if the indus-try price has become significantly discounted). This appears to be a straightforward comment, but it does raise two important issues regarding managerial accounting. Management needs to decide what costs are rele-vant to the decision at hand. That is, direct costs are often easy to identify, but how are overhead costs affected by the decision to accept a certain volume level? This is more difficult to determine. It also must be recog-nized that, in the short term, managers may not have much flexibility to alter their fixed costs. Therefore, only variable costs may be relevant to the pricing decision (i.e., to accept the offered price for services).

In contrast, health care organizations with relatively few competitors, large market shares, and leadership in the industry must decide what prices to set for their products/services. If the health care organization's products/ services can be differentiated from others because of enhanced quality, features, service, or other characteristics, the organization has more ability to set prices for them. Such health care providers are price-setters.

As a general decision rule, health care organizations that are price-setters (or price-setters for certain services/products) are in a position to make longer term pricing decisions when full costs are more relevant to the pric-ing decision at hand. These full costs include not only direct and variable costs but also proportionate burdens of the fixed cost structure and over-head. While such an approach to pricing strategy is desirable for all health care organizations (and, indeed, was basically facilitated by the regulatory environment), price-takers are not in a position to price on a full-cost basis.

It is important to recognize the fluid nature of the price-taker and the price-setter. These positions in the marketplace change regularly. For example, once two price-taker health care providers merge, they may become a price-setter as a merged entity. Also, organizations can have outstanding reputations for certain services and can command a premium to cover their full costs. For other services, however, they may be price-takers. Or, for the same service, the health care organization might be a price-taker in one geographical market and price more on marginal costs and a price-setter in another geographical market where it would price the service on more of a full-cost, premium basis.

Specific Issues Pertaining to Pricing Strategies for Health Care Services

One of the most significant changes in the health care industry in the past 20 years has been a dramatic shift in power from the seller to the buyer of health care services. Buyers are forming local coalitions to increase their financial leverage in negotiating with providers. Some would say that this shift means that revenues health care institutions receive will more and more be dictated by large purchasers of care—monopsonists and oligopsonists. These predominant purchasers of health care—HMOs, business coalitions, insurance companies, and government—have served notice that the marketplace is to be taken seriously in the dynamics that determine the prices of health care services. Furthermore, the seriousness of the marketplace as a formidable buyer is compounded by excess capacity in the health care industry. Dominant business coalitions can change the dynamics of pricing strategies of the health care organizations.

A final example of the seriousness of purchasers of health care services is reflected in the relationship between the auto industry and health care providers. The Big 3 automakers treat health care providers as they do suppliers of windshield wipers, batteries, and brakes, demanding top quality at the lowest cost and telling them exactly how to do it. These manufacturers are actively dispatching their productivity experts to their health care providers to improve productivity. This is important to auto manufacturers because the health bill for active and retired employees exceeds what these companies spend on a car's steel. Those outlays compare with minimal cost per car for the factories of some foreign automakers and almost zero cost for producers in countries with socialized medicine.

Among the concerns about the increasing strength of the buyer in the health care marketplace is the belief that these buyers, despite the rhetoric of cost and quality, will purchase exclusively on a low-cost basis. For example, one health care provider has outstanding mortality data for bypass surgery (1.4 percent). This excellent quality has been reflected in higher charges, with few discounts given to HMOs. The result has been that regional HMOs have chosen an alternative health care provider with higher mortality data that was among the earliest hospitals to agree to discount prices for HMOs. Similarly, another provider has attempted to market its reputation to health plans at higher prices, such as that for heart surgery, which is at least $2,000 above competition. This provider has been losing business to an alternative health care provider that has lackluster results (mortality rates) but continues to win discounted contracts from managed care plans.

According to many benefit managers, the market will become more consumer-driven because of the availability of increasingly useful outcome measurements. Certainly this demand for, and use of, quality information is at the heart of the logical purchasing coalitions. These groups achieve the goals of cost management and improved employee health care by being less prescriptive about health benefits and more proactive in demanding that health plans report better information about patient satisfaction, clinical outcomes, and overall value in delivering health-related services.

The increasing importance of quality in the consumer's decision to purchase health care services has been recognized by Standard & Poor and Moody's, which use quality assessments to determine hospitals' creditworthiness. These credit rating organizations feel that quality assessments are important because they demonstrate the stability of markets and demand forecasts and the ability to control resource use in times of declining reimbursement. For example, a quality measurement and management system helped one major health care provider obtain a double-A rating on a $90 million financing because it showed that the organization was positioning itself as a leader in documenting the quality of services it offered.

Many believe that deregulation and price competition in the health care industry will raise service quality and drive costly excess capacity out of the market, much as they have in the airline, trucking, banking, and railroad industries. Market competition has resulted in the end to managing hospitals as if they were country clubs, void of serious concerns for productivity and effectiveness. Although price elasticity of demand for hospital care is still relatively low, pricing decisions are still important to major purchasers.

Implications of Managed Care and the Assumption of Risk

Managed care covers a range of pricing philosophies: from fee-for-service, where the challenge is in setting discounts; to semi-flat rate such as DRGs and commercial product line pricing, where some risk is assumed by the provider; to full capitation that exposes the health care provider to significant risk if utilization goes unmanaged. For example, fee-for-service pricing essentially puts the provider at risk for only direct costs of service provision and levels of discounts offered. There is basically a positive incentive for the health care organization to utilize more resources at a micro-level (more tests, more procedures, etc.), keep the patient in the hospital more days, and admit more patients to the hospital. The only way the provider can be hurt in this payment arrangement is if net revenue after discounting the unit of service fails to exceed the direct costs of that unit of service. DRG payment, or the related commercial product line payment such as fixed-price contract for kidney transplants, now provides negative incentives for the hospital to increase utilization at the micro-level—resource by resource—and/or to increase days in the hospital. However, under this payment philosophy, it is still in the hospital's interest to maximize the number of hospital admissions pertaining to this DRG or commercial product line. Finally, the capitated payment philosophy provides negative incentives for the health care provider to maximize utilization across all three levels—at the micro-resource use, in terms of intensity, and in terms of encounters.

The whole focus of managed care systems as they move from fee-for-service toward capitation is to change the provider from a revenue center to a cost center. This focus becomes consistent with a target costing approach to pricing strategies in which the provider competes on competitive premium prices established in the marketplace and works backward to get its cost structure in line with market-defined prices. Part of the work on cost structure is dealt with by cascading health care services down to the lowest cost mode of delivery (e.g., moving away from the hospital) while maintaining quality. Essentially, the premium dollar has moved outside the hospital toward outpatient, nursing home, and home health care services. As a health care organization moves from fee-for-service to prepaid practice, the primary emphasis moves from revenue production to cost control.

Examples of moving away from a strict fee-for-service pricing strategy to a more risk-assuming strategy can be seen in the development of commercial DRG approaches in which the health care organization commits itself to a price for a defined diagnosis. For example, transplant centers are adapting pricing strategies based on fixed-price contracts that cover nearly all the expenses associated with organ transplants—cost of obtaining the organ, surgery fees, other hospital and physician charges, and a year of follow-up. To gain more HMO patients, these institutions are aggressively marketing their services in terms of these fixed-price strategies.

The switch to DRGs changed many hospital service departments from profit centers to cost centers but left the entire hospital as a profit center. Further movement toward fixed pricing, such as capitation payment, makes the hospital a service arm of a larger, more encompassing profit-making entity, the managed care enterprise. As a result of this change, the hospital's relationship to the organization changes from a producer to a consumer of revenues. And just as many health care organizations are adopting aggressive fixed-price strategies around product lines to win HMO patients, we also see health care providers adopting even more aggressive pricing strategies in terms of committing themselves to capitated revenues for defined populations. For example, one health care provider, in an unprecedented arrangement, agreed to provide comprehensive cancer care at a fixed price. This is the first contract of its kind in the cancer field. The provider receives a monthly fee per member in exchange for providing the HMO's patients with a full range of hospital, outpatient, and home care services. Similarly, another provider has signed a unique contract to provide oncological treatment under a capitated contract. The provider provides oncological treatment to the membership in one of only a few contracts nationwide in which oncology has been carved out. Some HMOs believe the method will help shift financial risk and rewards to other specialty medical organizations that try to deliver high-quality care at low cost.

The shift of risks will mandate that health care providers obtain access to better cost and utilization information. While cost and utilization data are important to the management of fee-for-service care, data are critical for a health care organization offering prepaid care. There will be increased scrutiny of what employees are getting for the employer's money, with development of data systems by the purchasers of health care that will match or exceed the information system of the health care organization. Buyers are seeking providers with feedback processes that can provide them with information and data documenting both clinical efficacy and cost efficiency. Health care providers might be advised to develop joint ventures with employers to build databases that can meet the growing demands of accountability. These data (market, financial, utilization, quality, and patient satisfaction) need to be collected and analyzed on a real-time basis. Effective contract negotiation requires that a hospital know its costs and whether the rate structure covers these costs and related margins.

The Roles of Budgeting in Health Care Organizations

Budgeting is an important part of planning a health care organization's economic activity. The budget is probably the most fundamental financial document in a health care organization and is most likely the first encounter that a health care manager has with accounting information. The organizational budget is a basic tool for tying together the planning and the control functions of management. More specifically, budgeting involves detailed plans, expressed in quantitative terms, that specify how resources will be acquired and used during a specified period. The predominant portion of this quantified plan is expressed in economic terms. Because many of these economic terms pertain to costs and revenues, budgeting applies much of our knowledge of cost accounting and pricing.

However, this quantified economic plan is not a detached analysis done by accountants. Derivation and use of the plan should infiltrate the entire organization. Thus, the budgeting process serves to facilitate communication and coordination throughout the organization. Each manager must be aware of plans made by other managers for the organization to be effective as a whole; essentially this process integrates the plans of each manager in an organization. Finally, the budgeting process and the resultant approved budget plan serve to allocate limited organizational resources among competing uses. These three major uses of the organizational budget—quantify economic plan, facilitate communication and coordination, and allocate organizational resources—are the front end of budgeting processes.

The richness and relevance of budgeting, however, is that it goes beyond planning, communicating, and allocating processes. There is also a back end to the budgeting process at which budgets are used in a feedback mode. That is, budgeting serves to help control operations and related profits. Plans are subject to change, and the budget serves as a useful benchmark within this change. Comparing actual results with budgeted results helps to evaluate the performance of individuals, departments, product lines, capitated contracts, etc. Because budgets are used to evaluate performance, they can also be used to provide incentives for people to perform well. Furthermore, information pertaining to what actually happened versus what was planned is incorporated into future plans to improve the accuracy of the planning process. The budget process forms a continuous loop of information—planning, implementing, controlling, and feedback.

It is important, in using the budget as an analytical tool, that analysis of variance between planned results and actual results is approached systematically. The starting point is the static budget, which is simply the original approved budget that has not been adjusted for differences between planned and actual volumes of services provided. The problem with static budgets is that they provide an expected cost, revenue, and profit for a particular volume, hence the name static. At the end of a reporting period, it is highly unlikely that we will have attained exactly the expected output level. If that is the case (as it almost always is), we end up with an apples-to-oranges comparison—for example, budgeted costs at one volume level and actual costs at another volume level. Based on the discussion of cost behavior, it should be obvious that, as the volume of patients rises, variable costs must rise. Just as obviously, if volume falls, we would expect that variable costs will fall. However, with the static budget, we do not know if the difference between budgeted and actual costs is due to different volumes of services or to some underlying inefficiencies.

To explain what is driving the total variance, we must move from a static budget to a flexible budget. A flexible budget is one in which the approved budget has been adjusted for volume changes. Essentially, flexible budgets are devices to tell what the results (revenues, costs, and profits) would be if a volume level was actually attained. The flexible budget approach places emphasis on the volume of patients actually treated by the organization (or, in the case of capitation, the volume of patients enrolled in the contract). The front-end of the budgeting process is very much like generating pro forma income statements. In preparing these budgets, we could prepare alternate budgets based on a range of possible volume outcomes. Each of these pro forma income statements could be considered to be a flexible budget based on the costs, revenues, and profits that we would expect to incur at a specified volume. The reason for different budgets at different volumes is that fee-for-service revenues should rise or fall with volume of services provided, capitated revenue should rise or fall with volume of enrollees, and variable costs should rise or fall with volume. This last point means that a flexible budget system must be developed on the basis of knowledge of which costs are fixed and which are variable.

Appendix C presents some basic budgeting techniques in both the static and flexible frameworks.

This concludes our introduction to the domain of financial and managerial accounting. In the next chapter we turn to the domain of managerial finance.

Endnote

*The relevant range of activity is typically the maximum capacity of the organization, using existing resources to deliver the service being analyzed within the period of time covered by the analysis. Should the provider decide to meet demand in excess of that capacity, additional capacity costs would have to be incurred. (Such additional costs themselves would almost always be fixed over the additional range of volume those costs would create.) In other words, no fixed cost is absolutely fixed.

Appendix A

Financial Statements

The financial statements produced by an accounting system contain information that can be critical in decision-making processes, especially those engaged in by top management and by parties external to the organization. Collectively, the various financial statements present the financial condition of the organization to management, stockholders, lenders, regulators, and other interested parties. Because, typically, the statements are prepared in accordance with generally accepted accounting principles (GAAP), the information can be analyzed and compared with that of previous years and, in some cases, with similar institutions. A thorough and continuing analysis of the financial statements can highlight potential problem areas and aid in determining corrective action.

Basic Financial Statements

The three primary types of financial statements are the balance sheet, the income statement, and the statement of "cash flow." Each of these statements has particular strengths and weaknesses for determining the financial condition of the organization.

The Balance Sheet

The balance sheet shows the financial position of the organization at a point in time. This can be the end of the year, the end of the month, or any other time desired by the administrator. Its reliability is determined by the accuracy of the accounting information and by the appropriateness of generally accepted accounting principles and regulations for the decision being made. The Financial Accounting Standards Board (FASB) and other professional accounting organizations issue guidance through pronouncements and opinions on appropriate accounting practices for presenting fair financial statements. For example, the physical assets of the organization are typically carried at their initial acquisition costs; the amounts carried in inventory and accounts receivable are a function of the accuracy of the record-keeping system and the time selected for the report. Some organizations will use the calendar year as their reporting period. Others may use another fiscal period that is more appropriate in terms of patient services and census. For example, a December 31 cutoff date for the balance sheet may have been selected more as a matter of tradition than because it is a proper time to analyze the financial position. December may typically be a low census month and some other time may be more representative. A typical balance sheet format and types of accounts are shown in figure A1, page 192.

Figure A1. Typical Balance Sheet

MEDICAL CENTER BALANCE SHEET—JUNE 30, 20x2 and 20x1

ASSETS	20x2	20x1
Current Assets:		
Cash and cash equivalents	$391,767	$1,125,628
Accounts receivable, net of allowance for uncollectible accounts and contractual allowances of $3,393,361 in 19x2 and $2,367,641 in 19x1.	8,399,210	7,524,313
Other accounts receivable	477,274	554,433
Reimbursement settlement receivable	72,601	80,668
Inventory of supplies	356,798	373,901
Prepaid expenses	53,251	80,714
Assets whose use is limited that are required for current liabilities	1,624,400	1,689,400
Total Current Assets	11,375,301	11,429,057
Assets whose use is limited by Board Designation		
Cash and cash equivalents	614,423	1,063,749
Short-term investments	6,348,645	2,966,819
Investment in pooled fund	1,842,483	2,551,979
Accrued interest receivable	31,628	10,079
Total assets whose use is limited	8,837,179	6,592,626
Less current portion	(1,624,400)	(1,689,400)
Net assets whose use is limited	7,212,779	4,903,226
Property, Plant and Equipment at cost:		
Hospital operations-		
Land and improvements	1,358,809	1,342,397
Buildings and leasehold improvements	16,607,453	15,556,408
Fixed equipment	14,206,950	14,209,592
Movable equipment	10,401,089	9,769,731
Other		
Construction in progress	80,170	768,910
Total property, plant and equipment	42,654,471	41,647,038
Less accumulated depreciation	(19,645,445)	(17,143,693)
Net property, plant and equipment	23,009,026	24,503,345
Deferred Professional Liability Costs	---	164,000
Deferred Financing Costs	533,517	587,313
TOTAL ASSETS	$42,130,623	$41,586,941

LIABILITIES AND FUND BALANCES	20x2	20x1
Current Liabilities		
Accounts payable	$2,326,397	$1,953,484
Accrued payroll, payroll taxes and employee benefits	2,000,348	1,900,659
Accrued interest payable	---	40,895
Other current liabilities	385,821	480,596
Reimbursement settlement payable	665,623	521,561
Payable to related division	630,000	---
Current portion of long-term debt	1,624,400	1,689,400
Total current liabilities	7,632,589	6,586,595
Other Liabilities and Deferred Revenue:		
Deferred revenue	70,560	72,240
Reserve for professional liability costs (Note 2)	82,000	164,000
Total other liabilities and deferred revenue	152,560	236,240
Long Term Debt		
Notes payable	13,949,900	16,354,300
Total long-term debt	13,949,900	16,354,300
Less-current portion	(1,624,400)	(1,689,400)
Net long-term debt	12,325,500	14,664,900
Commitments and Contingent Liabilities (Note 7)		
Fund Balances		
General	21,762,926	20,020,776
Restricted	257,048	78,430
Total fund balances	22,019,974	20,099,206
TOTAL LIABILITIES and FUND BALANCES	$42,130,623	$41,586,941

The components of the balance sheet are typically classified into definite groupings. For example, current assets include assets that are expected to be converted into cash or expenses within the current operating period or within one year. Assets limited as to use are internally restricted funds that have been identified by management for specific uses. The key term is "internally restricted"; the board can change either the amount or the classification. This can be contrasted to externally restricted funds, which require approval of the donor if changes in use are desired by management. Fixed assets are usually physical plant and equipment, which are expected to benefit more than one period. Fixed assets are converted into current expenses through depreciation techniques. The choice of depreciation methods can have a major impact on reported income and tax liability. Intangible assets are generally listed last because they are the least liquid of the assets and because their actual values depend on the provider's staying in business. Examples include deferred financing costs for debt that has been refinanced or attorney fees for reorganizational costs that have been incurred but must be expended over time because of GAAP.

Offsetting the asset accounts are liabilities and equity accounts of the organization. Liabilities consist of both short-term (current liabilities) and long-term (payable over more than one year) debt. Equity accounts are composed of the initial capital investment of the owners and the earnings retained in the organization from providing services. Equity accounts for not-for-profit organizations are sometimes called fund balances. The amounts reflect what has been retained in the organization after the amounts due to external creditors have been subtracted from total assets (total assets minus total debt equals equity/net worth/fund balances). Balance sheet accounts are usually considered to be permanent accounts; that is, they do not close at the end of each accounting period.

The Income Statement

The income statement measures the results of providing services over a period of time. It, too, is prepared in accordance with generally accepted accounting principles. The accrual method (matching of revenues and expenses), the depreciation method (straight line, accelerated), and the inventory valuation method can have a decided impact on reported income. Under the accrual method of accounting, and where noncash expenses such as depreciation are included, the income reported on the income statement is not the same as cash; in fact, using this method, it is possible to report high income and still experience a serious cash shortage. (This problem will be discussed in greater detail later in this section.) A typical income statement is shown in figure A2, page 194.

Figure A2. Typical Income Statement

MEDICAL CENTER		
Statement of Revenues and Expenses for the Years Ended June 30, 20x2 and 20x1		
	20x2	20x1
Operating Revenues:		
Net patient service revenue	$42,547,228	$40,075,756
Other operating revenue	1,131,716	1,085,983
Total operating revenues	43,678,944	41,161,739
Operating Expenses:		
Salaries and wages	18,417,626	16,742,397
Payroll taxes and benefits	3,422,329	2,992,994
Professional fees	2,161,173	1,811,640
Supplies and other expenses	12,546,593	12,456,113
Provision for bad debts	1,025,728	230,189
Depreciation and amortization	2,906,091	2,876,525
Interest expense	1,520,809	1,758,331
Total Operating Expenses	42,000,281	38,868,189
Income from Operations	1,678,663	2,293,550
Nonoperating Gains (Losses)		
Investment income, net	693,487	567,292
Other expenses	–	(90,000)
Total Nonoperating Revenues	693,487	477,292
Excess of Revenues over Expenses	$ 2,372,150	$ 2,770,842

The major components of the income statement are the revenue accounts and the expense accounts. The revenue accounts should be segregated by payer categories. The amounts shown as revenues do not include contractual allowances, discounts, and charity care. Only amounts that have been billed to payers will be included. Bad debts or amounts expected not to be collected are included as an expense account instead of as deduction from revenue. Charity care is only shown as a footnote to the summary statements and is no longer shown as a deduction from revenues. Nonpatient service revenues are shown as operating gains and losses after determination of net income from providing services to patients. Interest earned from investments would not typically be shown as patient care revenues and should be shown after net patient care income has been determined in order to correctly identify revenues earned from providing service to patients. In health maintenance organizations, interest earned can be shown as operating revenue.

Expenses are typically presented on a functional basis and reflect the amounts expended to provide the services responsible for the revenues shown in the income statement.

Income statement accounts are considered to be temporary accounts, because they are zeroed out at the end of each accounting period to prepare them for the next accounting period.

The Statement of Cash Flows

The balance sheet and the income statement have been required in annual reports for many years. In contrast, the statement of cash flows has only been required since the late 1980s. This relatively new financial statement has been added to the annual report in response to demands for better information about the firm's cash inflows and outflows. While the balance sheet provides a snapshot balance of cash of the final day of the period, it doesn't give the details of how it became that balance. A typed statement of cash flow is shown in figure A3, page 196. More specifically regarding Medical Center, for example, the unit of analysis for the statement of cash flows would be the difference between the ending cash balance of $391,767 and the beginning cash balance of $1,125,628 (a decrease of $733,861).

The statement of cash flows details how accrual entries on the income statement and changes in the accrual entries on the balance sheet (other than cash itself) relate to change in the cash position. The statement is intended to help the reader understand why and, to some degree, how the cash position decreased by $733,861. This change is not evident in the balance sheet by itself. And the income statement also tells only part of the story, in that net income is a major (but not the only) potential source of cash. That is, the net income of $2,372,150 may account for part of the increase in cash during the year. However, from a cash flow perspective, there are several adjustments to make to this net income figure before we can reach any conclusions as to the amount of cash contributed by operations. For example, as we had discussed earlier, we know that depreciation and amortization expense is a noncash expense. Thus, the cash generated from operations would be the $2,372,150 plus the depreciation expense of $2,906,091. However, there are other adjustments to be made to net income, such as recognizing that all revenue may not have been collected and all expenses may not have been paid. The details surrounding these adjustments are too complicated to cover in this chapter, but they are imbedded in the construction of the statement of cash flows.

Furthermore, cash may be raised by events not captured on the income statement. For example, the Medical Center may have raised cash by borrowing or by selling assets. Such events will be recognized in the statement of cash flows. Finally, even though cash increased from operations (with adjustments) and other sources, cash also went out. We do not see this on the income statement, but cash might have been spent to purchase assets or to pay off some debt. These are essentially transactions within the balance sheet that affect the cash position. These sorts of items would also be in the statement of cash flows.

Figure A3. Statements of Cash Flow

MEDICAL CENTER		
Statements of Cash Flow for the Years Ended June 30, 20x2 and 20x1		
	20x2	**20x1**
Cash Flows from Operating Activities:		
Excess of revenues over expenses	$ 2,372,150	$ 2,770,842
Adjustments to excess of revenues over expenses		
Depreciation and amortization	2,906,091	2,867,525
Bad Debt Expense	1,025,720	230,189
(Gain) Loss on sale of property, plant, and equipment	36,162	(19,346)
Restricted donations and grants	210,180	11,929
Expenditure of restricted donations and grants	31,622	(57,345)
Changes in operating assets and liabilities		
(Increase) decrease in:		
Accounts receivable	(1,900,617)	(1,808,847)
Other accounts receivable	77,159	33,131
Reimbursement settlement receivable	8,067	7,318
Inventory of supplies	17,103	(90,284)
Prepaid expenses	27,463	126,828
Deferred professional liability costs	164,000	(164,000)
Accounts payable	372,913	(303,320)
Accrued payroll, payroll taxes, and employee benefits	99,689	(33,391)
Accrued interest payable	(40,895)	(3,466)
Other current liabilities	(94,775)	(28,864)
Reimbursement settlement payable	144,062	521,561
Other liabilities & deferred revenues	(83,680)	162,320
Net cash provided by operating activities	**$5,309,170**	**$4,222,780**
Cash Flows from Investing Activities:		
Purchase of property, plant, and equipment	$(1,506,819)	$(2,814,626)
Proceeds from sale of property, plant, and equipment	112,741	29,499
Increase in assets whose use is limited	(2,244,553)	(337,626)
Net cash provided by investing activities	(3,638,631)	(3,122,753)
Cash Flows from Financing Activities:		
Principle payments on long-term debt	(2,404,400)	(1,285,400)
Increase in deferred financing costs		(17,550)
Net cash provided by financing activities	(2,404,400)	(1,302,950)
Net Decrease in Cash and Cash Equivalents	(733,861)	(202,923)
Cash and Cash Equivalents at Beginning of Year	1,125,628	1,328,551
Cash and Cash Equivalents at End of Year	$ 391,767	$ 1,125,628

In short, the statement of cash flows provides more valuable information about liquidity than can be obtained from the balance sheet and the income statement. The statement of cash flows shows where the health care organization generated its cash and how it used it over the entire period covered by the financial statement. This feature is similar to the income statement, which shows revenues and expenses for the entire accounting period.

However, the statement of cash flows is more encompassing than the income statement in that it also considers impacts other than from the income statement on cash flow (intra-balance sheet transactions), such as purchasing assets or retiring debt.

Therefore, the statement of cash flows is divided into three major sections:

- Cash from operations.
- Cash from/to investing activities.
- Cash from/to financing activities.

Operating activities are related to revenue- and expense-producing activities of the health care organization as reflected in the income statement. As stated above, these revenue- and expense-producing activities are adjusted by noncash amounts, such as depreciation expense, as well as several other more complicated adjustments. The working capital portion of the balance sheet is also considered among the ordinary activities of the firm, so changes in these amounts are also factored in. The financing activities of the health care organization are concerned with borrowing money (and repaying it), issuance of stock, and payment of dividends. All of these financing activities are potential non-income statement sources of cash (or drains on cash in terms of repaying debt or paying out dividends). Finally, the investing activities of the health care organization are also potential non–income statement uses of cash related to the purchase and sale of fixed assets and securities.

In summary, the income statement focuses on operations of the health care organization. Specifically, what did it cost to provide the service, what did it cost to operate the organization, and how much revenue did the organization get for its services? The statement of cash flows focuses on financial rather than operating aspects of the firm. Where did the money come from, and how did the health care organization spend it? While the major concern of the income statement is profitability, the statement of cash flows is very concerned with cash viability. Is the health care organization generating, and will it generate, enough cash to meet both short-term and long-term obligations?

Financial Statement Analysis

An analysis of financial statements can be accomplished by several methods. Single-point estimates can be obtained for comparison with other institutions or with external standards. A trend line is sometimes useful to identify possible problem areas. Both point and trend analysis are important for management information, but trend analysis has the added benefit of not requiring external comparison data. Because of the dissimilarity of

Figure A4. Summary of Ratios

Liquidity Ratios

Current Ratio	=	Current Assets / Current Liabilities
Daily Cash Outflow	=	Operating Expenses—Noncash Expenses / Days in Period
Days of Cash Outflow Available	=	Cash / Daily Cash Flow
Times Interest Coverage	=	Revenues in Excess of Expenses from Operations+ Interest Expense / Interest Expense
Debt Service Ratio	=	Revenues in Excess of Expenses from Operations + Interest + Depreciation + Annual Debt Service Requirements / Annual Debt Service
Working Capital per Bed	=	Working Capital / Available Beds

Turnover Ratios

Asset Turnover	=	Net Operating Revenue / Total Assets
Accounts Receivable Turnover	=	Net Operating Revenue / Net Accounts Receivable
Inventory Turnover	=	Supply Expense / Inventory
Average Daily Patient Revenue	=	Net Operating Revenue / Number of Days
Average Collection Period	=	Net Accounts Receivable / Average Daily Patient Revenue
Average Daily Operating Expenses	=	Operating Expenses / Number of Days
Accounts Payable Payment Period	=	Accounts Payable / Number of Days

Performance Ratios

Operating Margin	=	Revenues in Excess of Expenses from Operations / Net Revenues
Return on Assets	=	Revenues in Excess of Expenses from Operations / Total Assets
Return on Fund Balance	=	Revenues in Excess of Expenses from Operations / Fund Balance
Pre-Financing Return on Assets	=	Revenues in Excess of Expenses from Operations+ Interest / Total Assets
Pre-Financing Return on Fund Balance and Long Term Debt	=	Revenues in Excess of Expenses from Operations+ Interest / Fund Balance + Long-Term Debt

Capitalization Ratios

Total Debt to Fund Balance	=	Total Debt / Fund Balance
Long-Term Debt to Total Assets	=	Long-Term Debt / Total Assets
Total Debt to Total Capitalization	=	Total Debt / Total Assets

many institutions, point comparisons can be very misleading. The accounts in the balance sheet and the income statement can be analyzed on a percentage basis. Common size and vertical analysis provides information on changes in the structure of the statements in terms of percentages. These composition ratios can indicate when profit margins are shrinking and what is causing the decrease—for example, when certain asset categories are increasing in relationship to the total asset structure. An analysis of two statements is generally more effective than single estimates.

Another commonly used analysis technique is computation and comparison of ratios. Ratios can be grouped into specific management areas to aid in analysis. Four key management areas are:

Liquidity—Can the organization meet its current obligations?

Turnover—Are the organization's assets being used effectively?

Performance—Are the organization's assets being used efficiently?

Capitalization—How are the assets being financed?

A summary of the ratios is included in figure A4, page 198.

Sample Analysis of the Financial Statements

Using the data from figures A1, A2, and A3 and the ratios from figure A4, the following analysis could be accomplished for the sample provider:

Liquidity Ratios

Current Ratio $= \dfrac{11,375,301}{7,632,589} = 1.49$

Daily Cash Outflow $= \dfrac{42,000,281 - (2,906,091 + 1,025,720)}{365} = \$104,297$

Days of Cash Outflow Available $= \dfrac{391,767}{104,297} = 3.76 \text{ days}$

Times Interest Covered $= \dfrac{2,372,150 + 1,520,809}{1,520,809} = 2.56$

Analysis: The provider has a satisfactory current ratio, but the days of cash outflow are minimal. Collection of accounts receivable or short-term loans will be necessary to meet operating expenses.

Turnover Ratios

Asset Turnover $= \dfrac{43{,}678{,}944}{42{,}130{,}623} = 1.04$ times/year

Accounts Receivable Turnover $= \dfrac{43{,}678{,}944}{8{,}399{,}210} = 5.2$ times/year

Inventory Turnover $= \dfrac{12{,}546{,}593}{356{,}798} = 35.16$ days

Average Daily Revenue $= \dfrac{43{,}678{,}944}{365} = \$119{,}668$

Average Collection Period $= \dfrac{8{,}399{,}210}{119{,}668} = 70.19$ days

Average Daily Supply Expense $= \dfrac{12{,}546{,}593}{365} = \$34{,}374$

Accounts Payable Payment Period $= \dfrac{2{,}326{,}387}{34{,}374} = 67.68$ days

Analysis: Utilization of assets is average, as measured by the asset turnover of 1.04. The accounts receivable collection period of 70 days indicates some follow-up in this area would be useful, while the accounts payable cycle of 67.68 days means that bills are not paid promptly.

Performance Ratios

Operating Margin $= \dfrac{2{,}372{,}150}{43{,}678{,}944} = .054$

Return on Assets $= \dfrac{2{,}372{,}150}{42{,}130{,}623} = .0563$

Return on Fund Balance $= \dfrac{2{,}372{,}150}{22{,}019{,}974} = .1077$

Prefinancing Return on Assets $= \dfrac{2{,}372{,}150}{42{,}130{,}623} + 1{,}520{,}809 = .092$

Analysis: The owner has a reasonable operating margin (.054). The return on fund balance is high (10.77 percent) because of use of short-term credit in current liabilities.

Capitalization Ratios

Total Debt to
Fund Balances

$$= \frac{42{,}130{,}623 - 22{,}019{,}974}{22{,}019{,}974} = \frac{20{,}110{,}649}{22{,}019{,}974} = .91$$

Long-Term Debt
to Total Assets

$$= \frac{12{,}325{,}500}{42{,}130{,}623} = .29$$

Total Debt to
Total Assets

$$= \frac{42{,}130{,}623 - 22{,}019{,}974}{42{,}130{,}623} = \frac{20{,}110{,}649}{42{,}130{,}623} = .48$$

Analysis: The provider has 50 percent of capital from debt sources, which, in most cases, would be considered high. This may or may not be a problem, depending on the certainty of the payment process. If accounts receivable are sound, there should be no problem in paying off the debt. It might be prudent to add more long-term capital, through either retained earnings or a fund drive from the community.

Appendix B

Cost/Volume/Profit Models

Based on our understanding of cost behavior, a tool can be developed that will enable managers to make better forecasts of volume and better estimates of what the corresponding charge rate should be, or to assess more accurately the effects of changes in variable or fixed costs. To review our understanding of cost behavior, the following definitions are presented:

- Variable costs are assumed to vary directly in proportion to the volume of services provided.
- Fixed costs are assumed not to vary with volume changes.

Given these two basic assumptions, the cost structure for the service can be expressed as follows:

(1)   Total Costs (TC) = Total Fixed Costs (TFC) + Total Variable Costs (TVC); TC = TFC + TVC.

(2)   TVC = Variable Costs per Unit of Service (VCU) x Volume (or number of units) of Service (Q). Therefore, equation (1) can also be expressed as TC = TFC + (VCU x Q).

(3)   Average Total Cost (ATC) = Total Cost per unit x Volume of service = $\dfrac{TC}{Q}$

The first three equations can be expressed in the following model when revenues and profits requirements are introduced:

(4)   Total Revenues (TR)[1] = Rate per Unit of Service (R) x Volume of Service (Q); TR = R x Q.

Desired Profit or Income (I) can be expressed as a dollar requirement or as a percentage of total revenue requirement and on a before- or after-tax basis.[2]

(5a) After-tax dollar requirement = I
      Before-tax dollar requirement = I/(1 - tax rate)

(5b) After-tax percentage of total revenue requirement = %TR
      Before-tax percentage of total revenue requirement = %TR/(1 - tax rate)

The summary and complete model can be expressed as:

(6) $TR = TC + I$ or

$R \times Q = TFC + (VCU)(Q) + I (1 - \text{tax rate})$

or, solving for R,

(7) $R = \dfrac{TFC}{Q} + VCU + \dfrac{I}{(1 - \text{tax rate}) \times Q}$

An example of how this equation can be used is to determine the rate that must be charged to obtain a desired level of profit.

Given:

TFC	=	$50,000
VCU	=	$11
Desired Income (after taxes)	=	$10,000
Tax rate	=	37.5%
Q	=	5,000

Substituting:

$R = \dfrac{\$50,000}{5,000} + 11 + \dfrac{\$10,000}{(1 - .375) \times 5,000}$

$R = \$10 + 11 + \dfrac{2}{(1 - .375)}$

$R = \$10 + \$11 + \$3.20 = \$24.20$

This answer can be verified by completing a simplified income statement:

Total Revenue	5,000	x	$24.20	=	$121,000
Variable Costs	5,000	x	$11.00	=	$ 55,000
Contribution Margin	5,000	x	$13.20	=	$ 66,000

Total Fixed Costs	$ 50,000
Income Before Taxes	$ 16,000
Taxes at a $37^{1/2}$ % Rate	$ 6,000
Income After Taxes	$ 10,000

The basic cost/volume/profit model of equation (7) can also be used, for example, to compare the effects of buying more equipment (increased fixed costs) with those of switching to outside suppliers on a fee-for-service basis (increased variable costs). Of course, the estimates going into the model do not have to be, indeed cannot be, precise. Few events in the future can be determined precisely. What is needed is an estimate of the reasonableness of the numbers. Is this rate reasonable? Can this quantity realistically be obtained? How sensitive are the results to alternative assumptions? The model allows the input necessary for this type of analysis.

Capitation

The basic cost/volume/profit model of equation (7) can also be used in a capitated environment. However, the volume factor (Q) must be expressed in the manner in which we generate revenue—the monthly premium dollar that is referred to as member months (mm). In this case, let us assume that we are considering a contract to cover 125,000 mm. Thus, Q = 125,000 mm. The unit of service expression from the fee-for-service example (5,000) is still relevant. Instead of the volume factor (Q), however, it is a utilization expression. Thus, utilization (U) = 5,000 units ÷ 125,000 = .04 per mm. At this point we can set the price (monthly premium) that we need to achieve the desired income of $10,000 as expressed in the fee-for-service environment. This is done in the following:

Given:

TFC	=	$50,000
VCU	=	$11
Desired Income (after taxes)	=	$10,000
Tax rate	=	37.5%
Q	=	125,000
U	=	.04 mm

Substitutions:

$$R = \frac{\$50,000}{125,000 \text{ mm}} + \$11(.04) + \frac{\$10,000}{(1-.375) \times 125,000 \text{ mm}}$$

$$R = .40 \text{ mm} + .44 \text{ mm} + .128 \text{ mm} = \$.968 \text{ mm}$$

This answer can be verified by completing a simplified income statement:

Total Revenue	125,000 mm	x	.968	=	$121,000
Variable Costs	125,000 mm	x	.44	=	55,000
Contribution Margin	125,000 mm	x	.528	=	66,000

Total Fixed Costs	$ 50,000
Income Before Taxes	16,000
Taxes @ 37.5% Rate	$ 6,000
Income after Taxes	$ 10,000

Following this logic further, notice the positive implications if we are able to control utilization such that it drops from .04 mm to .03 mm. This results in variable costs being expressed as .03 x $11 unit = $.33 mm. These implications are seen in the following simplified income statement.

Total Revenue	125,000 mm	x	.968	=	$121,000
Variable Costs	125,000 mm	x	.33	=	41,250
Contribution Margin	125,000 mm	x	.638	=	79,750
Total Fixed Costs					50,000
Income Before Taxes					29,750
Taxes @ 37.5% Rate					11,156
Income after Taxes					$ 18,594

Note this improvement in income: $18,594 – 10,000 = $ 8,594. This increase results from control of utilization as follows: .01 (decrease in utilization from .04 to .03) x $11 x 125,000 mm = $13,750 less $5,156 (the 37.5 percent tax rate) = $8,594.

Multiple Payers

For many departments, there is no single rate for services provided because of the varying amounts paid by different third-party payers. Each individual rate may reflect third-party regulations; competitive pressures; and/or managerial judgments about future costs, market dynamics, inflation, etc. Once individual rates have been estimated, the same approach described above can be used, but the single rate used in the model above becomes a weighted average of the various payer rates. In the example above, a single rate of $24.20 resulted. But this $24.20 could represent an average rate developed in the following manner:

	Proportion of Total Volume	x	Rate		
Medicare	30%	x	$20.00	=	$ 6.00
Medicaid	50%	x	15.40	=	$ 7.70
Charge-Based	20%	x	52.50	=	$10.50
		Average Revenue		=	$24.20

The following example shows how the rate for a charge-based payer can be determined where multiple payers exist.

Given:

- 40,000 lab tests are forecast.
- The Medicare rate is $32.00 and Medicare is 40% of all activity.
- The Medicaid rate is $20.00 and Medicaid is 50% of all activity.
- Charge-based activity is 10% of all activity.
- Fixed costs are $600,000.
- Variable costs are $10.00 per lab test.
- The desired profit margin is $100,000 after taxes.
- The tax rate is 37.5%

What rate must be charged to charge-based payers to meet the desired profit margin? Using the model developed above and substituting the new information, the average rate would be:

$$RA = [TFC + (VCU \times Q) + \frac{I}{(1 - \text{tax rate})}] \div Q$$

$$RA = [\$600,000 + (\$10 \times 40,000) + \frac{\$100,000}{(1 - .375)}] \div 40,000$$

$$RA = \frac{\$600,000}{40,000} + \$10 + \frac{\$160,000}{40,000} = \$15 + \$10 + \$4 = \$29$$

Using the weighted average approach developed above, the charge for charge-based payers would be:

	Proportion of Total Volume	x	Rate		
Medicare	40%	x	$32.00	=	$ 10.00
Medicaid	50%	x	20.00	=	$ 12.80
Charge-Based	10%	x	RChg	=	$?
		Average Revenue		=	$29.00

RChg = ($29.00 - $10.00 - $12.80) divided by .10 = $6.20 ÷ .10 = $62.00, the required charge for charge-based payers.

These results can be verified using the income statement approach:

Revenues

Medicare	40%	x	40,000	x	$32.00	=	$ 512,000
Medicaid	50%	x	40,000	x	22.00	=	400,000
Charge-Based	10%	x	40,000	x	62.00	=	248,000
			Total Revenue				= $1,160,000

Expenses

Fixed Costs	$ 600,000
Variable Costs (40,000 x $10)	400,000
Total Costs	$1,000,000
Profit before taxes	$ 160,000
Taxes at 37.5%	60,000
Profit after taxes	$ 100,000

If the mix of the various payers changes, the effect on the rate can also be determined and adjustments can be made accordingly.

A Contribution Model

A short-cut approach to the cost/volume/profit model is one that focuses on the contribution margin (CM) or on the difference between the rate (R) and the variable cost per unit (VCU). Through concentration on the contribution margin, answers can rapidly be obtained to the questions posed above. For example, the basic contribution model can be expressed as:

$$(8) \qquad TFC \quad + \frac{I}{1 - \text{tax rate}} = Q \times CM$$

where I is the desired after-tax income and CM is defined as (R - VCU).

Given the numbers in the first example above:

R	=	$ 24.20
TFC	=	$50,000
VCU	=	$ 11
I	=	10,000
Tax rate	=	37.5%
Q	=	Unknown

Substituting in the Equation (8):

$$\$50,000 + \frac{\$10,000}{(1 - .375)} = Q \times \$13.20$$

$$Q = \frac{\$50,000 + \$16,000}{\$13.20}$$

$$= \frac{\$66,000}{\$13.20}$$

$$= 5,000$$

The contribution margin approach can also be used effectively to monitor and report on departmental activities. The basic format changes to define margin as the difference between total revenues and direct costs (TR - DC). Direct costs include all costs for which the department supervisor is responsible. For example, the department supervisor is responsible for salaries paid and supplies used. Depreciation on equipment used only in the department, any special maintenance, etc. are considered direct costs. Other costs, such as general administration, utilities, and housekeeping, are considered indirect costs, because they are not under the control of the department supervisor but are generally allocated. An example performance report might be:

Total Revenues	$100,000
Total Direct Costs	70,000
Direct Margin	$30,000
Allocated Indirect Costs	25,000
Departmental Income	$5,000

The direct margin should be the point of emphasis for the control process. The amount of indirect costs can be changed by the choice of allocation methods as well as by third-party payment regulations. Although the bottom line is a proper concern of senior managers, it is questionable whether it should be used to evaluate lower levels of supervisors, whose range of choice and control is limited.

Footnotes

1. Total revenues are defined as the amount expected to be collected from all patients.

2. This works for not-for-profit organizations as well. With a tax rate of zero, the before-tax and after-tax requirements are simply equal.

Appendix C

Basic Budgeting Techniques

Flexible and Static Budgeting

Identification of variable and fixed cost components of cost categories makes it possible to use flexible budgeting techniques. A flexible budget is a budget that is adjusted for volume changes. For example, if nurse staffing is based on patient days, the budget allowance for nurse staffing would change with changes in patient activity level. Nursing administration costs, in comparison, are relatively fixed for reasonable ranges of patient activity.

Suppose 65,700 patient days were budgeted for a hospital's revenue projections. If we required 2.5 RN hours per patient day, our budgeted RN hours would be 65,700 x 2.5 = 164,250. These hours could then be converted to a dollar cost by extending them at the average RN hourly rate. If that were $12 per hour, the total budgeted cost would be $1,971,000. If we did not adjust this budgeted amount for variation in patient days, we would be using a static budget approach. The budget logic is as follows:

	Output	Standards	Input
Budget	65,700 days x	2.5 RN hours = per day	164,250 RN hours $12 $1,971,000

A static budget approach to making judgments about organizational performance would take the planned budget as the basis against which to compare actual RN salary costs during the period. This adherence to a budgeted amount when costs are variable can lead to dysfunctional managerial decisions. For example, if patient days are less than planned, the budget for RN salaries would be too loose, and, even if actual RN costs were equal or slightly less than the budgeted amount, RNs would not have been used efficiently. If patient days are greater than planned, strict adherence to the budgeted RN costs would result in fewer RN hours being available for each patient day, and a reduction in the quality of care could result.

Flexible budgeting adjusts the budget for changes in levels of activity. For example, assume actual nursing costs were $2,203,200. Also assume that the number of patient days was 68,000, compared to the 65,700 that were planned. A static budget suggests an unfavorable variance:

	Output	**Standards**	**Input**
Budget	65,700 days x	2.5 RN hours = per day	164,250 RN hours x $12 $1,971,000
Actual	68,000 days x	2.7 RN hours = per day	183,600 RN hours x $12 $2,203,200

Unfavorable Variance   (1,971,000 – 2,203,200) $(232,200)

However, a flexible budget would first adjust expected cash to the actual value level before determining the variance:

	Output	**Standards**	**Input**
Budget	65,700 days x	2.5 RN hours = per day	164,250 RN hours x $12 $1,971,000
Flexible Budget	68,000 days x	2.5 RN hours = per day	170,000 RN hours x $12 $2,040,000
Actual	68,000 days x	2.7 RN hours = per day	183,600 RN hours x $12 $2,203,200

Total Variance   ($1,971,000 – 2,203,200) $(232,200)

Volume (allowable) ($1,971,000 – 2,040,000) $69,000
(2,300 additional patient days x 2.5 RN hrs/day x $12)

Unfavorable Variance ($2,040,000 – 2,203,200)$(163,200)

In most organizations, the flexible budget approach offers a more realistic assessment of performance and a better approach to cost control. For many providers, when most costs are relatively fixed, the static budget approach may be adequate. But if variable costs, even if relatively small, can be determined, the flexible approach provides more detailed information and can identify excess as well as insufficient resource utilization.

Hugh W. Long, MBA, PhD, JD, is a Professor of Health Systems Management in Tulane University's School of Public Health and Tropical Medicine. He holds additional appointments at Tulane's School of Law and its Freeman School of Business and is a member of Tulane's Graduate School faculty. He is the founder of the first Master of Medical Management program.

Mark D. Covaleski, PhD, CPA, is Professor of Health Care Financial Management at the University of Wisconsin-Madison. He is also adjunct faculty member of the Department of Health Systems Management at Tulane University and teaches in its Master of Medical Management program.

Chapter 11

Fiscal Management of Provider Organizations: Part II

by Hugh W. Long, MBA, PhD, JD
and Mark Covaleski, PhD, CPA

Finance

The introduction to Chapter 10 presented the basic concept that the domain of finance focuses on matters quite different from those addressed by financial accounting, and of longer horizon than those addressed by managerial accounting. While managerial accounting is clearly focused on the future, the future it addresses is typically short-term. Financial accounting primarily deals with reporting an organization's historical activity in fiscal terms and secondarily makes forecasts of future financial statements and performance. Managerial accounting, while to a large extent breaking from the structures of financial accounting, still tends to focus on accrual concepts. Further, managerial finance, in contrast to financial accounting, is exclusively future-oriented and, in contrast to managerial accounting, deals with fiscal decision making on sources of financing and resource allocation (uses of financing) over the full range of time horizons. Both accounting and finance make important contributions to managerial processes, but they are very different from each other.

For example, while accrual accounting tries to match dollar figures with physical events, such as "patients served," finance matches dollar figures only with fiscal events, such as the collection of monies for services to patients. As a result, finance is concerned with the accounting accrual concept in only peripheral ways. Finance focuses not on when service delivery occurs but rather on when money associated with that service comes in or goes out the door. Are you going to collect tomorrow, next week, or two months from now? Are you ever going to collect? When does the cash flow occur? Similarly, finance does not associate resource cost with the timing of resource use, but rather with the timing of the payment for the resource.

Finance focuses on receipts, not revenue, and on expenditures, not expenses. This is because it is concerned with future cash flows or their equivalents, not past performance, and because, ultimately, only cash matters in capital markets.

Suppose that you order a diagnostic laboratory test today that is performed today and a corresponding charge is generated at the same time. Assume further that medical supplies already on hand were used to obtain and to test the specimen. An accrual system will recognize the revenues from the test today, whether or not any collection occurred today. If there was no collection, the accrual system will recognize a corresponding increase in "accounts receivable" on the balance sheet. Finance will recognize nothing until the actual collection occurs. The accrual system will also recognize the "expense" of the supplies today, reducing an "inventory" (of supplies) account on the balance sheet. Finance will recognize nothing today unless there is a cash outlay today for those supplies.[1] Finance is interested in and will recognize only actual cash inflows and outflows, regardless of when the economic activity that gives rise to those flows takes place.

Finance also treats capital expenditures very differently from how they are treated by accounting. If you decide to spend $100,000 for a piece of equipment that is expected to be productive for five years, the $100,000 is gone as soon as you acquire the equipment. Finance "recognizes" the full "outlay" of the equipment when the cash outflow for the equipment takes place. It does not matter if the machine is going to last two years, five years, or 10 years.

The financial accountant will record the expense of the equipment in installments during which the equipment is used. Each installment will be labeled "depreciation expense" and will appear on an income statement covering some part of the time the equipment is being used. The amounts of each installment will reflect various rules and formulas, but will not themselves reflect any cash outflows in those amounts. For this reason, depreciation expense is not, by itself, relevant to finance. Finance pays attention to depreciation expense only if its presence affects some other cash flow, for example, tax payments.

Why does finance place all of its emphasis on cash flows? Because finance focuses on the organization's ability to command resources (goods and services) and capital and its ability to service its capital in the future. At root, these abilities rely directly on the use of cash, of money.

Money is like any other resource, in that an organization must pay for the privilege of using it. Examples include paying interest on a loan or on a bond issue (debt financing), distributing profits (dividends) to partners (stockholders) for profit (equity financing), or providing charity care and supporting teaching and research (not-for-profit equity financing). The organization's ability to make such "rent" payments, plus its ability to repatriate the capital itself directly, affects whether or not it will be able to attract future capital.

Buying resources and servicing capital ultimately requires cash. You cannot meet next Friday's payroll with accounts receivable, revenue, or even income (all accounting measures). You can only meet the payroll with cash or its equivalent, e.g., checks drawn against bank balances. This is why decision making, analysis, and evaluation in finance look at the ability of the organization to meet next Friday's payroll, to buy supplies next month, and to service its capital into the indefinite future— i.e., to generate required levels of cash flow. You can defer some things in the short term by borrowing money, of course, but, ultimately, you must have the cash to repay the borrowing. Thus, while you can shift future cash flows around in time, at some point you finally get to the economic bottom line requiring cash in the bank.

In identifying organizational cash flows, finance focuses on incremental analysis, because it is analyzing the future for the specific purpose of assisting managers in making decisions. That is, finance considers only changes in cash flows that may result from a decision. Should we buy a new computer for the accounting department? Finance analysis will look at the timing and amounts of cash outflows and inflows only to the extent that they differ from what they might be if the new computer is not purchased.

In finance, the time value of money is always explicit.[2] A dollar today is always different from a dollar tomorrow. If you try to add a January dollar to a December dollar, you are doing what your second grade teacher told you never to do: You are adding apples and oranges. From an economic point of view, January and December dollars are not the same thing, partly because the effect of inflation causes their purchasing power to differ. They are also not the same thing for a variety of other reasons having nothing whatsoever to do with purchasing power. Even if a dollar in January bought the same quantity of real goods and services as a dollar would in December, (i.e., there was no inflation or deflation), you would not be indifferent to the choice between these two time-separated dollars. If you receive a choice between a dollar's worth of purchasing power today and a dollar's worth of purchasing power a year from now, you would still choose the dollar today rather than the purchasing-power-adjusted dollar a year from today. If nothing else, you could always take the dollar today and invest it at a risk-free real (after-inflation) investment rate of two or three percent. That two or three percent represents the compensation required to induce people to defer consumption of real resources.

The finance function includes:

- Constructing forecasts of distinct sets of future cash flows, each associated with alternative courses of organizational action.
- Establishing valuation criteria based on estimates of required rates of return.[3]
- Using those criteria to evaluate the relative worth of alternative sets of future cash flows.
- Assisting managers in integrating this economic information into decision-making and planning processes.

Finance forecasts and evaluations are primarily designed for internal, managerial purposes rather than for outside parties. They are not to be relied upon for external applications or as a vehicle for the implementation of public policy as are the outputs of accounting. They are an input to decision-making and planning processes, primarily internal.

There are several broad categories of decisions that are amenable to analysis from a finance perspective:

- Decisions focused on near-term cash flows, so-called "working capital management."
- Capital structure decisions.
- Capital acquisition and disbursement decisions.
- Long-term investment/divestment choices, so-called "capital budgeting" decisions.[4]

The first three of these areas are largely the province of the controller/CFO/treasurer of the organization, while the fourth area is more the province of operational managers supported by the fiscal function. Management of the organization's near-term cash inflows and outflows addresses questions such as: "How much cash should we keep in the bank?" "How big should our inventories be?" "What should our policy be on charging interest on past due accounts?" "What's our collection policy?" "How fast should we pay our bills?" "Should we invest in Treasury bills?" "Should we prepay insurance premiums?" Working capital management decisions are generally based on how variable the organization's cash flows are and on what effect the choices have on an organization's ability to meet its required rate(s) of return.

Capital structure matters are another decision area to which the health care industry has historically paid little attention. Few organizations have explicit policy positions on the mix of debt and equity that finances their assets and programs. For each organization, there is some particular capital structure range that offers optimal cost and risk characteristics, and, typically, that structure includes significant quantities of debt and/or lease financing.

Capital acquisition and disbursement decisions address raising and servicing capital. This is different from the capital structure decision, which concerns the proportions of debt and equity capital used by an organization. Capital acquisition, by contrast, deals with how you plan to bring capital into the organization as cash (or, in the case of leasing, as real assets). Capital disbursement involves planning for what goes back out the door as cash or in-kind dividend payments, salary "bonuses" to owners, other distributions of accounting income, and interest and principal payments on debt. For debt capital, should we have level debt service, balloon payments, declining debt service? For equity capital, how much should we retain, how much should we repatriate? Correctly structured, these types of transactions ensure organizational continuity, both in being able to provide health services and in having needed access to capital markets.

The "capital budgeting decision" encompasses all decisions involving the initiation and/or the abandonment of programs and services and the resultant retention and/or the termination of personnel. Should we acquire this equipment, initiate this new service, hire this physician, sell off this part of the business, close this department, not replace persons at retirement? How do we structure a portfolio of assets, people, and programs?

In all four categories of decisions just described, finance provides the economic component, the projection of what will best enable the organization to meet or exceed its capital suppliers' required rates of return, thereby preserving or enhancing organizational value. That is what finance is all about.

The Changing Role of the Chief Financial Officer

In the 1960s, the health care industry had very little competent financial management. Indeed, the state of fiscal management in most health care provider organizations, if it existed at all, was roughly comparable to the level of fiscal sophistication in the rest of American industry in the 1870s. In prior decades, when most health care providers in the private sector were largely supported by philanthropy and public-sector grants and when health care costs were not an item of major national policy concern, fiscal management beyond simple bookkeeping and occasional audits was seen largely as a luxury.

It was only after the advent of the major national entitlement programs, Medicare and Medicaid, that the majority of health care providers instituted double-entry accrual accounting. In the years since 1966, the health care industry developed highly competent financial accounting and, since the advent of Medicare's Prospective Payment System and the rise of prepaid health care in the 1980s and 1990s, has added sophisticated cost accounting. In addition to financial accounting and cost accounting, managerial accounting, especially in the areas of budgeting and control, has also become the managerial standard. What remain in the process of adoption, however, are finance techniques that have been at the forefront of fiscal management for the rest of American industry since shortly after World War II, techniques of such import that they were the basis for two Nobel prizes in economics awarded during the 1990s.[5]

Thus, while today's CFO is light years away from the green-eyeshade bookkeeper who ran the business office of the 1940s and 1950s, he or she is still more likely to use pro forma financial statements and/or a cost accounting approach than one involving net present value (a finance method discussed later in this chapter) and much more likely to rely on balance sheet information on organizational value than to build alternative systems to estimate market values directly. The key to sound fiscal management is to appreciate the strengths and weaknesses of all of these approaches to resource allocation, to appreciate the interrelationships between fiscal and nonfiscal elements within an organization, and to communicate broadly within the organization, speaking not in "fiscal" tongues but in common language.

Value: Measurement, Maintenance, Enhancement

This section introduces the following concepts of finance:

- Debt and Equity Capital
- Rate of Return
      "Pure" interest or "the time value of money"
      Adjustment for expected inflation
      Business risk
      Adjustment for taxation
      Interest rate risk

- Financial Risk and Capital Structure
- Cost of Capital and Weighted Average Cost of Capital
- Net Present Value

These concepts and the techniques related to them form the foundations for financial evaluation. They are used to evaluate an organization's current financial status and to evaluate what effect, if any, a given proposal or course of action will have on that financial status. The underlying normative principle of finance is that each discrete organizational activity should at least "pay for itself," because if too many activities are "losers" (without offsetting "winners"), the organization will eventually find its survival threatened. Finance is also quite pragmatic. It recognizes that there are times when activities should be supported even though they are not fiscally viable by themselves, if the organization is capable of providing that support. For example, professional personnel might be encouraged to teach at local universities or do research in clinical areas. For these purposes, they receive release time or its equivalent. From a financial perspective, this policy has a direct, measurable cost and no associated measurable income. Yet there is little doubt that the professionals' participation in such activities benefits the organization's reputation.

The point is that finance always focuses on the measurable economic consequences of an organization's actions. This analysis is, of course, only one input, although certainly a very important one, to the organization's decision-making and planning processes.

Debt and Equity Capital

The economic foundation of any private-sector organization (in the health care field or in any other industry) is its capital. That capital, whatever its mix of debt and equity, supports the entire structure of assets owned (or resources controlled) and programs engaged in by the organization. The ultimate success, indeed the very survival, of the organization depends on the extent to which its utilization of assets and program activities provides fiscal returns sufficient to preserve and/or enhance the underlying capital base.

Preserving and enhancing capital is a fundamental task of any organization in the private sector. Within the private sector, of course, we have both for-profit and not-for-profit organizations. We may characterize not-for-profit organizations as entities that should, at minimum, preserve (maintain) the economic value of their capital, while for-profit organizations need to go the further step of enhancing the economic value of their capital.

For-profit organizations are created to increase the wealth of their owners. This can happen in two ways. First, economic profits can be returned to the owners in cash. Second, profits can be reinvested in the organization, which increases the market value of owners' equity. In accounting terms, equity is literally the extent to which the value of all organizational assets exceeds the value of all organizational liabilities (debts). In the real (financial) world, owners' equity is the market value of owners' claim on the organization if they wished to sell those claims to a willing buyer.

In the not-for-profit case, "owners" are considered to be parent entities, the community, or the public at large. The return to the community is the services that the organization provides and its ability to continue to provide those services over time. As good stewards, managers of not-for-profit organizations must also attempt to make an accounting profit (i.e., to have revenues exceed expenses).[6] But how large a profit and what the organization does with it are entirely different questions. For example, a not-for-profit provider having a "profit" in a given year might choose to use the portion that a for-profit counterpart might use for dividends or owner wealth enhancing investment to:

- Lower its charges (or simply hold them constant while competitors' rates go up).

- Offer additional services in non-income-producing areas, such as health education, support of research, or additional charity or deeply discounted care.

- Retain and invest monies in relatively liquid, low-risk assets, helping to carry the organization through lean times.

- Replace or add real assets to improve the quality of or access to services provided.

The key concept here is that all organizations must show an accounting profit (have revenues greater than expenses) if they are to survive in the long run.[7] This is equally true of not-for-profit and for-profit firms. What distinguishes the two is what is done with the profit, if any, that exceeds the amount needed to preserve capital.

Preservation of Capital

The term "preservation of capital" has a very specific economic meaning. What we wish to preserve or maintain is the real value of capital, the claims of the existing suppliers of the fiscal resources supporting the activities of the organization. Because capital comes from an external, competitive marketplace, the ability to satisfy those who have, in the past, supplied capital is the key element to being able to attract new capital from those or other suppliers in the future.

Satisfying capital suppliers means meeting their expectations. All suppliers of capital to the private sector expect some form of return in exchange for their having supplied the capital, and those expectations exist whether the capital was supplied to a for-profit or a not-for-profit organization.

Suppliers of debt capital are readily identified as institutions and individuals having contractual claims against the organization—for example, a commercial bank that has extended credit, an insurance company holding a mortgage, a pension fund holding a private placement of bonds, or individuals holding bonds that were publicly offered. The expectations of suppliers of debt capital as to returns are clear and explicit. They are embodied in the contractual terms agreed to in advance by themselves and the borrowing organization in a loan agreement, mortgage contract, bond indenture, or the like.

Most suppliers of equity capital to a for-profit organization are clearly identifiable. Shareholders of a corporation, the partners in a partnership, or the owner of a sole proprietorship supply equity capital to those organizations. For the not-for-profit health care provider, equity suppliers are somewhat more diverse and, other than when it is the wholly owned subsidiary of a parent not-for-profit entity (e.g., a religious organization), more difficult to identify individually. The list may include private donors of cash, be they major philanthropists, private foundations, or persons contributing a few dollars to an annual fund drive; volunteers who provide wage and salary expense relief to the institution or program; payers of tax monies that flow through a government entity to the provider by grant, appropriation, or designation[8]; and a small number of recipients of health services who, themselves or via third parties, pay more than the economic cost for those services. Because of the breadth and the diversity of these equity capital suppliers, we generally refer to them as "society," "the community," or "the service area."

There is, of course, no written contract concerning specific returns to suppliers of ordinary equity capital. Further financial accounting deliberately excludes all reference to returns on equity capital as an expense (unlike the recognition by financial accounting of interest expense, the return on debt capital). As a result, managers (even of for-profit firms) sometimes fall into the trap of viewing equity capital as free, as having no explicit cost, that is, requiring no returns. Nothing could be further from economic reality.

The shareholders or the partners of a for-profit organization have very clear expectations of dividends or cash distributions and/or appreciation in the market value of their ownership claims. Suppliers of equity capital to not-for-profit organizations also have specific expectations of return. The fact that these returns are not permitted to be in the form of cash distributions or market value appreciation in no way lessens the strength of the expectations or reduces the economic burden on management to meet those expectations. Suppliers of equity capital to not-for-profit health care providers expect those organizations to remain viable into the indefinite future[9]; they expect the social value of the services provided by such organizations to exceed the organizations' charges for providing those services; they expect such organizations to support, as appropriate, relevant educational programs and research; and they expect reasonable levels of free and/or discounted care to be provided to certain segments of the community served. Indeed, the range of equity supplier expectations may be quite large.

Required Rate of Return

The rate of return required by any supplier of capital will, of course, vary through time. A generic rate of return conceptually includes compensation for five major factors, any one of which can change at any time in a dynamic marketplace:

- The pure "time value of money"
- Inflation (deflation)
- Default
- Untimely/forced liquidation
- Expected taxation

The pure time value of money is simply economic recognition that consumption of goods and services has positive value to human beings and, because of the finite lifespan of human beings, cannot be postponed indefinitely. Individuals, directly and through the organizations they form, draw satisfaction from consumption[10] and require compensation for anything that delays that consumption. That is, because we prefer to consume sooner rather than later and because supplying capital to others effectively delays the supplier's ability to use those funds for consumption, a "pure rate of interest" is required to compensate for the delay. Empirically, the pure rate of interest as an annual rate has been in the 2 to 2.5 percent range.

For example, suppose a bank supplies $36,000 of capital to an organization today and expects the loan to be paid back after one year. The bank may require (expect) $828 (2.3 percent) worth of compensation one year from now in recognition of the fact that the bank's money has been tied up for one year. Thus, a payment to the bank of $36,828 one year hence would provide a full return of and on capital.[11]

The second component of a required rate of return is the additional compensation necessary in an inflationary environment to compensate the capital supplier for expected loss of purchasing power. (In the case of expected deflation, an adjustment reducing the overall required rate of return would occur.) Between the time the capital is initially supplied and the time that returns to capital are made, price increases in the capital supplier's "market basket" of goods and services will have reduced the real value of the supplier's initial investment. The purchasing power adjustment that compensates for this expected loss of value is applied both to the initial capital itself and to the compensation-for-delayed-consumption (pure interest) return.

Continuing the numerical example begun above, if a 4 percent inflation rate is expected (that is, it will take $10.40 one year from now to buy the same quantities of goods and services now costing $10.00), the bank would require payment of $38,301.12 one year hence ($36,828 plus 4 percent of $36,828).

The third component of an overall required rate of return on capital is compensation for the risk of possible nonpayment or delay in payment of some or all of the total return due to the capital supplier.[12] Default arises because of an insufficiency of cash to service capital, reflecting cash flow variability that derives primarily from an organization's basic economic activity (business risk). For each class of capital supplier, the risk can be mitigated or magnified by the relative position (priority or lack thereof) of that class's claim among all capital claims on the organization (financial risk).[13] Financial risk and its implications will be considered in more detail in the next section. Business risk arises from the nature of the economic environment and from operational characteristics of each organization.

One way to think about business risk is to array three categories of elements: systemic risk (inter- and intrasystem phenomena—e.g., political factors such as expropriation or nationalization of assets—fluctuations in exchange rates, monetary and fiscal policy), market risk (e.g., elements of competition, public and/or private regulation, supplier power, third-party purchasing power, technological obsolescence), and organizational risk (e.g., quality of managerial and operating personnel and processes, input/output efficiency). All of these elements interacting will cause some organizations to experience cash flows that fall short of what is required to meet the expectations of some or all of their capital suppliers, with a resultant default.

It is important to recognize the differential roles of management in addressing these three categories of risk. Managers have virtually no control with regard to systemic risk. Managers may be able to exert only some influence on various elements of market risk, through, for example, negotiations with suppliers or purchasers. But managers are largely responsible for the decisions that define the level of organizational risk.

Continuing our numerical example begun above, suppose that the bank expects a one percent rate of complete default (i.e., for every 100 loans of this type made, 99 are paid in full on time, and 1 goes to total default and repays nothing). To cover this contingency, the bank will charge a premium on each loan it makes. To compute the premium, divide the total payment that fully compensates the bank for the pure time value of money and for inflation by one minus the failure rate:

$38,301.12/(1-.01) = $38,301.12/.99 = $38,688.00

This assures the bank of full returns on all of its loans by spreading the risk of failure across all the loans it makes:

100 x $38,301.12 = $3,830,112 = 99 x 38,688.00

Other, slightly more complicated calculations are possible that would take into account partial repayments and late repayments.

The fourth component of a basic rate of return deals with the generic risks associated with an uncertain future. Suppliers of capital, like all managers, attempt to forecast future economic conditions. Good as our crystal balls and computer models may be, no one can have absolute confidence in forecasts of next year's monetary policy, inflation rate, and rates of taxation or of the likelihood of default on a claim. Thus, required rates of return fluctuate daily, as expectations about future events and conditions change. In this fluctuating environment, the capital supplier bears the risks associated with the possible necessity of having to sell the capital claim for an unknown price[14] to someone else prior to its original or expected maturity. The further in the future the expected maturity, the greater is the possibility of having to do this. Not only is there the possibility of sustaining a capital loss, but generally there will also be conversion or transaction costs associated with the untimely or forced liquidation of the claim.

These risks of loss are in part related to the amount of time remaining until all returns to a capital claim are expected to be realized—the longer the time, the greater the risk—but they are also related to the natural degree of volatility in the claim-specific risk factors noted above and to the efficiency or lack thereof in the secondary market for the claim. Typically, an additional premium for bearing such risks, an "illiquidity premium,"[15] is observable in required rates of return as compensation for future interest rate (and capital value) fluctuation. While there is no way to calculate an exact amount for the illiquidity premium, it might be as little as one-half of one percent for a one-year maturity and several percentage points for a 10-year maturity.

In our example, rather than requiring $38,688.00, the bank might ask for an additional $193.44 (a one-half of one percent), or a total of $38,881.44.

The fifth component of marketplace required rates of return is compensation for taxation. Different taxes may be levied simultaneously by several different levels of government, and the nature and rate of taxation levied by each level may depend on the characteristics of both the supplier and the user of the capital.

Suppose, in our example, that the return on the $36,000 in capital (that is, all return in excess of $36,000, or $2,881.44) is considered taxable income. Because that $2,881.44 is seen as what is necessary to fairly compensate the capital supplier for real interest, inflation, the risk of default, and the risk of untimely liquidation, the capital supplier must receive before-tax compensation of sufficient magnitude so that after meeting the tax liability, $2,881.44 will remain. To find the appropriate before-tax amount, simply divide the required after-tax dollar return on capital by one minus the applicable marginal tax rate. If the bank in this example had to pay tax at a marginal rate of 27.5 percent,[16] the required payment would be:

$36,000 + $2,881.44/(1−.275) = $36,000 + $2,881.44/0.725 = $36,000 + 3,974.40 = $39,974.40, or an 11.04 percent required rate of return.

The capital marketplace brings together suppliers and users of capital representing the full spectrum of different tax and inflation environments, all manner of sensitivities to risks, and widely divergent opinions as to future economic conditions and business risks. Hence, market-determined rates of return ultimately represent the relative supplies of and demands for capital from many heterogeneous market participants. Nonetheless, market-clearing rates of return necessarily satisfy capital suppliers in the conceptual dimensions noted. If they did not, the capital would not be supplied.

Classes of Capital Suppliers, Financial Risk, and Required Rates

The discussion above of required rates of return was generic for all suppliers of capital. The simplest capital structure is that of an organization with no debt and a single owner (equity), while complex capital structures may contain several types of debt, a number of categories of equity, and various forms of leasing. For this section we consider only the first level of complexity—an organization having just two kinds of suppliers of capital, both internally homogeneous: suppliers of equity capital and suppliers of debt capital.

Although debt suppliers may not have been the first parties chronologically to provide capital to the organization, they are definitely the parties first in line to receive returns to capital. This is because organizations enter into explicit contracts with suppliers of debt, promising to pay them specific sums of interest and principal at definite future times. These contractual claims take precedence over returns to equity suppliers, who are legally entitled only to whatever is left after all contractual claims are fully satisfied.

Therefore, debt is always viewed as less risky than equity, because debt has first claim on the organization's cash flows. There is, therefore, a difference in the financial risk faced by suppliers of debt and equity capital.

If an organization were 100 percent equity-financed, equity would bear all of the risks and costs discussed earlier. If the organization approached being 100 percent debt-financed, debt would have assumed almost all of these risks and costs. At points in the middle (say 50 percent debt and 50 percent equity), debt's first claim on the organization's resources makes it less risky than equity, and thus its required rate of return will be less. Indeed, debt's risk is not only less than equity's, but also is less than the average risk of the overall organization.

In a parallel manner, equity's inherent risk would be magnified by the financial risk associated with increasing proportions of debt having a priority claim in the capital structure. As debt claims a greater and greater share of operational cash flows available to service capital, it becomes increasingly likely that variability in those flows might leave little or no funds after debt service to meet the expectations of equity suppliers. Equity suppliers require a higher rate of return to compensate them for bearing this financial risk over and above the other risks and costs. If there is any debt at all, equity's required rate of return will be higher than debt's and higher than the average rate of return for the overall organization. At high levels of debt financing, equity holders might well require annual rates of return in the 30-40 percent range.

The Cost of Capital

Up to this point, required rates of return have been discussed primarily from the perspective of the capital supplier. The other side of the coin, of course, is the cost of capital to the user. In the simplest cases, these are identical. What the capital supplier receives is what it costs the organization. Various circumstances, however, can cause the cost of debt service to the organization to be less than the required rate of return actually received by the capital supplier.

For example, a corporate for-profit provider pays taxes on its net income, taxable revenues less deductible expenses. Interest is one such deductible expense. Suppose a for-profit provider paying taxes at a rate of 40 percent decides to borrow $1000 for one year at an interest rate (required rate of return) of 10 percent. The loan will accrue $100 of interest expense at the end of the year. If the borrower would have had $500 of taxable income without the borrowing, taxes due would have been $200 [=40 percent of $500]. With the borrowing, taxable income is now $400 [=$500 - $100 interest expense] and taxes due are now only $160 [=40 percent of 400]. The tax bill has declined by $40 from $200 to $160. Hence, the $100 interest expense has been partially offset by the $40 tax savings, leaving a net cost for the borrowing of $60. That net cost of $60 is 6 percent of the $1,000 borrowed. Even though the lender receives its full required rate of return of 10 percent ($100), the cost to the borrower is only 6 percent ($60). The 4 percent ($40) difference is, in effect, a government subsidy to the borrower. It lowers the cost of debt to the organization because a third party is absorbing a portion of the return actually received by the capital supplier.[17]

The basic point is that the economics of producing returns to capital (the costs of capital) need to be distinguished from the returns themselves (as viewed by the capital suppliers receiving them).

The long-run survival of any private sector organization, for-profit or not-for-profit, depends on its ability to renew existing capital (not assets) and to attract new capital from time to time. This ability to succeed in attracting infusions of capital from an increasingly competitive capital market relates specifically to the organization's demonstrated ability to preserve the real economic value of existing capital. That value is preserved only if each class of capital supplier receives its respective required rate of return. Because parts of that required rate of return may be provided (or reduced) by external parties (e.g., taxation authorities), internal organizational decisions need to focus only on the net cost of capital. Thus, a provider's operational fiscal returns must attain the cost of capital threshold so that, when supplemented (or reduced) by external parties, capital suppliers will receive their required rates of return and be willing to renew or expand their provision of capital to the organization.

Meeting the expectations of some but not all capital suppliers is insufficient. For example, paying all of the contractual interest and principal payments on time is not, by itself, enough to guarantee future access to capital. It is also necessary to preserve the value of equity capital in order to maintain a strong overall capital structure. A weak equity position is just as surely a hindrance to future borrowing as is failure to meet debt service payments.

Selection of Organization Activities

The "bottom line" (both figuratively and literally) of financial analysis is determining whether or not a given organizational activity (e.g., opening a new clinic, adding more physicians, buying a computer, adding a new service) will pay for itself in the long run or be a drain on the organization's resources (i.e., equity). To do this, finance computes the weighted average cost of capital; identifies the incremental operational cash flows associated with the activity; and, from them, determines the net present value of the alternative or activity.

An organization obtains capital from many different sources: bank loans, individual investors or contributors, grants, bond issues, etc. Each source will have an associated cost of capital. One useful statistic for financial analysis, therefore, is the "weighted average cost of capital" (WACC). This is simply the cost of capital for each supplier weighted by its proportion of total capital measured at market value. For example, suppose a provider is financed by (has total capital of) $1,000,000[18]: a $250,000 loan and a tax-exempt bond issue for $500,000 at net (after-tax and after-reimbursement) costs of 10 percent and 7 percent, respectively, and a $250,000 infusion of equity from a parent entity requiring a 12 percent rate of return. The WACC of this organization would be:

$$\underbrace{\frac{250{,}000}{1{,}000{,}000} \times .10}_{(\text{Loan})} + \underbrace{\frac{500{,}000}{1{,}000{,}000} \times 0.07}_{(\text{Bond})} + \underbrace{\frac{250{,}000}{1{,}000{,}000} \times .12}_{(\text{Equity})} =$$

$$0.25 \times 0.10 + 0.50 \times 0.07 + 0.25 \times 0.12 = 0.025 + 0.035 + 0.030 = 9.00\%$$

Second, the incremental, operational cash flows associated with the activity must be identified. Operational cash flows are nonaccrual measures of all the cash flows in and out of the organization other than cash flows to and from capital suppliers (e.g., interest payments) and cash flows triggered by capital supplier flows (e.g., tax reductions in recognition of interest payments). Operational cash flows, therefore, exclude equity infusions and dividends but include inflows from asset liquidation and outflows for asset acquisition.

In addition to the requirement that cash flows be of the operational rather than the capital type, they also must be strictly incremental. This simply means that we count only those cash flows that will change as a result of the decision regarding the proposal under consideration.[19]

Fiscal evaluation of any proposal begins with an estimate of the expected incremental operational cash flows associated with the proposal, period by period, over an appropriate future time. Once this stream of cash flows is obtained, it must be evaluated in terms of the organization's WACC. This is because organizations should focus on their costs of capital rather than on capital's required rate of return. Specifically, the WACC is used as the "rate of discount" with which to find the value today of a proposal's expected incremental future operational cash flows (including the proposal's expected investment outlays now and henceforth). This value today is called the proposal's net present value (NPV). A positive NPV means that a proposal pays for itself (including the cost of capital to support it) and that there will be funds left over that can be put to other uses. An NPV of zero means that a proposal breaks even in economic terms; it will pay for itself but generate no additional resources beyond the required returns. A negative NPV means that the organization will have to subsidize the proposal, because it cannot be economically self-supporting.[20]

Calculating a proposal's NPV using the WACC as the discount rate involves determining the relative value of each of the incremental operational cash flows.

For all the reasons discussed earlier, as long as there is a positive rate of return, a dollar in hand today is more valuable than a dollar expected tomorrow. If a 20 percent annual rate of return is required (or available), one dollar invested today at that rate will be worth $1.20 one year hence. Similarly, one dollar expected a year from now is worth only 83 1/3 cents today.[21] The discount factor (1.20 in these examples) is equal to one plus the appropriate discount rate expressed as a decimal.

Because the calculation of NPV is largely mechanical,[22] we won't go into great detail here, but a simplified numerical example in the Appendix to this chapter illustrates the application of this concept of value measurement. Net present value is a powerful concept that allows comparison of different courses of action and their consequences in economic terms. However, it is important to remember that financial evaluation is just one input into the overall decision-making process.

Some Normative Considerations

Positive-NPV activities increase an organization's value (i.e., the value of its equity) even after all suppliers of capital, including equity, are satisfied, in the sense of having received exactly their required rates of return. The increase in value in today's dollars is equal to the positive amount of NPV. Negative-NPV activities show the amount by which the value of the organization will decline in today's dollars if all required rates of return are met. (Meeting such requirements is accomplished by drawing down the value of existing equity, a process in which many providers engage, often unknowingly.) In the long term, of course, organizations with negative-NPV portfolios cease to exist through one of two mechanisms. In the most severe case, termination by bankruptcy occurs. In the milder circumstance, future access to the capital markets is denied and a less traumatic liquidation or sale or merger occurs.

For-profit providers have an economic obligation to maximize the wealth of their ownership, subject to all the usual legal and ethical constraints. Hence, for-profit providers should actively seek as many positive-NPV activities in their portfolio of assets and programs as possible.

By contrast, not-for-profit providers should be seen as having an overall neutral-NPV portfolio of activities. This in no way precludes the growth of the organization, for it says nothing about the number or size of activities engaged in. Rather, the "rule" is that not-for-profit organizations should seek an overall portfolio of activities that achieves only a small positive NPV, meeting the required rates of return of all capital suppliers and relevant community constituencies.

For example, consider the example of a hospital or a clinic that is considering a new marketing program that (it is predicted) will have a highly positive NPV. A for-profit organization might choose to increase dividends or distributions to equity as the new income is realized, or it might choose to reinvest the "extra" dollars in activities that increase owners' equity. A not-for-profit organization is faced with the same question: What do we do with the extra dollars? It might choose to add a health education program (return of social value to community); support clinical research or teaching (return to community) and probably an "in-kind" or noncash bonus to workers (increasing the organization's viability); reduce prices to some patients or provide additional charity care (social dividend); or simply retain the money as liquid, short-term assets, such as CDs or Treasury bills (increase organization viability).

A negative-NPV proposal, by definition, is incapable of sustaining itself economically. Assuming all possible cost efficiencies have been incorporated in the proposal, the only way to adjust the value of such a proposal upward is to increase its operational cash inflows by posting higher prices (rates). If, ultimately, such increases are constrained by competition, rate regulation, ordinary price elasticity in the marketplace, or other economic or political factors, and the NPV still remains negative, the proposal must be rejected as a "mainframe" (nondividend)[23] activity. However, this does not necessarily mean that the proposal should be rejected totally. Financial analysis using NPV is only one input into overall decision making. Besides economic factors, there are two other generic concerns that must be examined: long-run strategic payoffs and "social" value.

At this point, the organization's board should review such uneconomic proposals (assuming they are of sufficient magnitude to warrant such attention). The substance of the proposal (e.g., the actual service to be delivered) may be viewed by the board as so important to the community that the board will declare the activity a dividend (to the community)[24] or so integrally intertwined with the organization's mission that it is considered essential. Neither step should be taken lightly (which, of course, is why the matter should be brought to the board in the first place).

Take the case of a social dividend to the community. If the provider is currently meeting the expectations of its equity capital suppliers, does not offset the new dividend by a reduction in an existing dividend, and wishes to maintain the current value of its capital (i.e., does not wish to partially liquidate through a return of capital), the board, by declaring the dividend, is saying the community expects (requires) the dividend as part of its overall return. This simply means that, unless new inflows of equity capital can be found, mainframe activities will have to bear the additional cost of the new dividend, thereby implying price increases.

If the cash inflows from existing mainframe activities cannot be increased (again assuming cost efficiency has already been attained) and new equity capital is not forthcoming, the dividend that has been declared is, in effect, a partial liquidating dividend. There is absolutely nothing wrong with declaring a partial liquidating dividend, of course, as long as it is done consciously, explicitly. Adopting negative-NPV projects (effective dividends) without being aware of their long-run economic implications, however, can clearly endanger long-run organizational survival.

With respect to strategic decisions to invest in "essential" activities, it is important that organizational decision making and board policy formulation take a long-run perspective if the organization is to remain viable in a dynamic and competitive environment. On the other hand, the factors cited above (cross-subsidization and partial liquidation of capital) also need to be considered. This approach to explicit, board-level formulation of dividend policy has the major advantage of bringing issues of cross-subsidization out of the shadows and placing them on top of the table for direct deliberation and decision making.

Finally, all organizations should attempt to minimize their WACCs. For a given set of programs and activities, a lower WACC will clearly generate more wealth for for-profit ownership and greater price reductions in the not-for-profit sector. Additionally, more proposals will have NPVs greater than or equal to zero, thereby allowing a broader range of both mainframe services and dividends.

Techniques for minimizing WACC are among a number of advanced fiscal management subjects that cannot be addressed in detail here, but they would include determining and implementing an optimal capital structure, taking a wide variety of possible actions to minimize perceived business risk, and ensuring that the lowest cost sources of capital are being tapped. It is worth noting that the latter technique is one of the stronger economic arguments for retaining tax-exempt debt financing for not-for-profit providers. The lower WACC that results from tax-exempt financing also permits the broader range of mainframe services and dividends noted above.

Summarizing Finance and Accounting

As we have seen in this and the previous chapter, finance and accounting are important functional areas within the discipline of management.

Financial accounting focuses on ex post reporting to internal and external parties and helps managers assess the recent past performance and the current fiscal position of the organization.

Managerial accounting is integral to the understanding of cost structures, cost behavior, pricing, and operational budgeting. Some managerial accounting deals with attributing long-run resource costs to individual units of output. Other facets of managerial accounting focus on operational budgeting.

Both financial and managerial accounting have particular processes and formats through which information is generated, reported, and analyzed. For ex post reporting, there are income statements, balance sheets, and statements of "cash flow" that are generated by double-entry accounting systems applying generally accepted accounting principles. Managerial accounting uses various models and tools to analyze and manage costs, and, like finance, encompasses a variety of analytical techniques that focus on the future. Unlike finance, managerial accounting focuses more on the day-to-day functioning of the provider and relatively short future horizons extending out one to two years.

Finance is primarily concerned with assisting managers in making resource allocation and financing decisions that are consistent with economic value criteria. Finance focuses on forecasting future fiscal events and on evaluating alternative forecasts against value criteria tailored to each organization. Finance, too, has special models and protocols, and is generally concerned with the longer-term future extending over the entire life cycles of assets or financing vehicles that could extend for 10 or 20 or even 30 years.

Further Study of Finance and Accounting

To appreciate fully the range of finance and accounting concepts and tools requires much more study than we have been able to cover here. Well-rounded physician executives need to achieve a level of understanding of these concepts and tools well beyond the scope of these chapters, and excellent starting points for anyone wishing to go more deeply into such material appear in the bibliographic entries following the appendix to this chapter.

We have provided some very brief comments about each entry, but as a more general proposition for both these and other sources, exercise caution in using the title of such books as a reliable indicator of the actual contents. For example, just because the word "finance" or "financial" appears in the title of a work does not tell you whether that reference is about accounting or finance.

Endnotes

1. If the supplies were paid for at an earlier time, finance would have noted the outlay at that time; if the supplies are not yet paid for, a debt (liability) has been incurred, and finance will recognize the future outlay as a reduction of debt.

2. When relatively small amounts of money are involved for relatively short periods of time during which market rates of return—e.g., interest—are relatively low, the quantum of time value is relatively small. It is for this reason that managerial accounting, typically dealing with only a year or so of the future, generally dispenses with incorporating time value into its analyses.

3. Organizations must service their capital to include paying "rent" on the money/resources they use in providing their health care service or product. But how much rent must be paid? Capital suppliers (whether debt or equity) will require a certain rate of return on their funds. In an analogous manner, the organization must also achieve a certain rate of return when it allocates these capital resources to one use or another. Thus, finance has as one of its most basic and important functions ascertaining the appropriate rates of return an organization must (on average) attain from the goods and services it provides in order to achieve long-run economic survival.

4. This is actually a misnomer, because the subject matter in this decision category involves neither capital nor budgeting.

5. The 1990 Nobel Memorial Prize in Economic Science was shared by Harry Markowitx, William Sharpe, and Merton Miller for their work in financial markets and corporate finance. Robert Merton and Myron Scholes shared the same award in 1997.

6. To illustrate why a bottom line (net income) that is literally zero is unacceptable—indeed, on an income statement, why a small positive bottom line may also be inadequate—consider the following: If your investment advisor had you invest $100,000 on January 1 for one year and you received a check the following December 31 for $102,000 for the full liquidation of your investment, you would have a $2,000 bottom line, a $2,000 accounting profit (and, if you were a taxable entity, you would owe taxes on that $2,000). You would also be looking for a new investment advisor, because, notwithstanding your "profitable" year, you are less wealthy at December 31 than you were the previous January 1, because, if for no other reason, $102,000 will buy less December 31 than $100,000 would have a year earlier as a result of normal price increases.

7. Having an accounting profit is a necessary but not a sufficient condition to ensure survival. As shown in endnote #20, an organization with a positive bottom line on its income statement may still be failing economically.

8. In addition to direct subsidies, there are indirect subsidies, as, for example, the granting of tax-exempt status and the right to issue tax-exempt securities, both of which tend to raise others' taxes and to make up for the government revenue shortfalls ("tax expenditures") thus created. Another indirect subsidy is the income-tax deductibility of contributions to 501(c)(3) organizations.

9. The accountant embodies this expectation in applying the "ongoing enterprise" principle; the attorney does the same thing in referring to the corporation as "an infinite-life individual" under the law.

10. Consumption is broadly defined here to encompass not only the acquisition of services and material goods but also charitable activity from which the donor derives satisfaction.

11. Return of capital is exactly what it sounds like: the organization pays back money it has been supplied. This is the case when we pay off the principal portion of the loan. Return on capital is the "rent" paid for the use of the money, as, for example, the interest portion of a loan payment. The combination of returns of and on capital is called return to capital.

12. The so-called "risk-free rate," which is the required rate of return on federal government Treasury securities, is a rate that contemplates no risk of default. This is because the federal government literally can't default, because the government could always manufacture the money that its securities promise to pay. The risk-free rate, however, recognizes that such securities have all of the other four factors that require compensation.

13. E.g., employees get paid before suppliers, suppliers get paid before bondholders, secured debt gets paid off before unsecured debt, debt gets paid off before equity holders receive any distributions.

14. Or even a known price in the case of a discretionary call or a random mandatory call by the organization to which the capital was supplied.

15. One sometimes hears the term "liquidity premium." This refers to the higher price the market typically (but not always) places on claims with short-term maturities. Because prices and rates of return are inversely related, the terms "illiquidity premium" or "duration premium" refer to the usually higher rates (lower price) on longer time-to-maturity claims.

16. This assumes that there are no offsetting incremental deductions for expenses. If there were, they would lessen the tax burden.

17. It is also possible to have a lower cost of capital in other ways. For example, a not-for-profit provider may also be able to pay interest that is nontaxable to the lender, thereby lowering its cost of capital by choice of financing vehicle. (Tax-free bonds are the most common example of this type of arrangement.) This mechanism, however, does not cause a difference between the organization's cost of capital and the capital supplier's required rate of return, because it simply lowers both.

18. In WACC computations, market values of debt and equity claims are always used rather than "book" or accounting values.

19. One circumstance to be careful of occurs when the adoption of a proposal obviates a future operational cash flow otherwise required in the absence of favorable consideration afforded the proposal under consideration. For example, suppose a room would need to be repainted next year. A proposal to institute a new service this year calls for complete renovation of this space now, dispensing with the cost of repainting the room next year. For the purpose of analyzing the proposal, the cost of painting the room next year is treated as a relevant, incremental, operational cash inflow next year associated with the new service proposal. This is because the proposal saves money that would otherwise have been spent.

20. Note that a proposal that generates positive net income as measured by GAAP may have a negative NPV. For example, suppose a provider invests $210,000 for one year and at the end of the year receives back $216,300, a 3 percent rate of return and an accounting profit of $6,300 (3% of 210,000 = $6,300; $210,000 + $6,300 = $216,300). If the required rate of return on the $210,000 of capital were 5 percent, however, this investment would have an NPV of ($4,000), a negative value. [See Appendix; $216,000/(1.05) = $206,000; $206,000 - $210,000 = ($4,000)] Incidentally, that negative $4,000 is also the present value of the shortfall between what was actually received at the end of the year, $216,000, and what would have been received had the required rate of return been achieved: 5 percent of $210,000 = $10,500; $210,000 + $10,500 = $220,500; $216,300 - $220,500 = ($4,200); ($4,200)/(1.05) = ($4,000). The point here is that, although the investment has positive net income under GAAP, it is not sufficiently profitable to provide all capital suppliers their required rates of return. If this proposal were characteristic of the resource allocation decisions being made by the managers of the provider organization, it would be viewed by capital suppliers as unsatisfactory employment of their capital, and they would refuse to make future capital infusions. When that refusal causes the provider to have to forgo investments that are requisite to organizational survival, the provider will disappear, the discipline of the capital markets having prevailed.

21. $0.83\frac{1}{3}$ return of capital plus $0.16\frac{2}{3}$ return on capital (20 percent of $0.83\frac{1}{3}$), equals a $1.00 total return.

22. Many pocket calculators are preprogrammed to perform a number of simple present value calculations, and all basic spreadsheet software for personal computers includes present value functions.

23. A "mainframe" activity is one that is economically self-supporting, a "tub on its own bottom" not requiring external or cross-subsidization to exist. Mainframe activities are those meeting the WACC criterion, thereby providing the cash flows needed to service the organization's capital.

24. Depending on corporate philosophy, for-profit as well as not-for-profit providers may choose widely different approaches to community dividends. The not-for-profit "community-owned" provider, of course, has a much more direct economic tie to its service area and typically must meet higher expectations regarding returns to equity capital in the form of in-kind dividends than the for-profit provider, which also returns cash to the community in the form of taxes.

Appendix

Net Present Value Calculations

Assume that a proposal to be evaluated requires an initial cash investment of $1,000 and is expected to provide incremental cash inflows of $372 at the end of the first year and $1,296 at the end of the second year. The organization's overall WACC is estimated to be 20 percent during both years. This 20 percent rate means that the $1,000 investment should provide a total return of at least $1,200 if the proposed activity lasts just one year. But this proposal covers two years, and, while it provides only $372 in the first year, it also generates $1,296 in the second year. This means that we must evaluate both of the cash inflows to see if their combined value provides a total return sufficient to meet our 20 percent WACC.

To value flows over two years, we simply do what we already know how to do, but we do it twice:

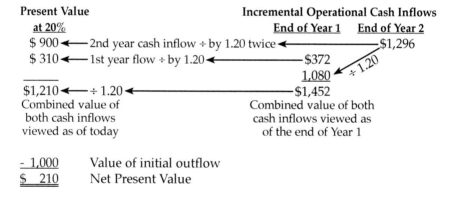

Present Value at 20%	Incremental Operational Cash Inflows

$ 900 ←— 2nd year cash inflow ÷ by 1.20 twice ←————— $1,296
$ 310 ←— 1st year flow ÷ by 1.20 ←————— $372
_____   1,080 ÷ 1.20
$1,210 ←— ÷ 1.20 ←————————————————— $1,452
Combined value of   Combined value of both
 both cash inflows   cash inflows viewed as
viewed as of today   of the end of Year 1

- 1,000   Value of initial outflow
$ 210   Net Present Value

Because the present value of the $1,000 initial cash outflow today is a negative $1,000, the NPV of this proposal is a positive $210. Obviously, this proposal is very desirable from a fiscal viewpoint.

A different way of arriving at the same result is as follows:

1. $1,000 invested at 20 percent for two years yields $1,440 = ($1,000 x 1.20 x 1.20). Therefore, if a proposal returned exactly $1,440 on a $1,000 investment after two years it would exactly meet the organization's WACC and have a net present value of zero.

2. But this proposal returns $372 after one year and $1,296 the second year. Because they're not the "same" kind of dollars, you can't just add $372 and $1,296. But you can adjust the $372 by presuming you could invest it at the same 20 percent rate that was applied above:

$372 x 1.20 = $ 446.40   (value of first year payment at end of second year)

1,296.00   (Second year payment)

$1,742.40   (Total return at end of second year;
also the combined value of both cash inflows
viewed as of end of year 2)

3. Comparing the $1,742 total return after two years to the $1,440 required return from Step 1, the proposal generates extra return of $302.40. This amount is called the "net future value" of the proposal.

4. To convert net future value to net present value, you have to discount it back for two years. As discussed previously, you simply divide the $302.40 by the discount factor (in this case 1.20) twice, because two years of adjustment have to be made: $302.40 ÷ 1.20 = $252.00; $252.00 ÷ 1.20 = $210.00, the net present value calculated initially.

Hugh W. Long, MBA, PhD, JD, is a Professor of Health Systems Management in Tulane University's School of Public Health and Tropical Medicine. He holds additional appointments at Tulane's School of Law and its Freeman School of Business and is a member of Tulane's Graduate School faculty. He is the founder of the first Master of Medical Management program.

Mark D. Covaleski, PhD, CPA, is Professor of Health Care Financial Management at the University of Wisconsin-Madison. He is also adjunct faculty member of the Department of Health Systems Management at Tulane University and teaches in its Master of Medical Management program.

Chapter 12

Physicians & Health Care Organizations as Co-Fiduciaries of Patients:
A Key Concept for the Ethics of Physician Leadership

by Frank A. Chervenak, MD, MMM, CPE, FACPE
and Laurence B. McCullough, PhD

The concept of physicians and health care organizations as co-fiduciaries of patients is of vital importance at this time.[1,2] Being a fiduciary of patients means that:

- One possesses expert knowledge and skills about how to protect and promote the health-related interests of patients.
- One is committed to using that expertise primarily for the benefit of the patient and to making self-interest a systematically secondary consideration.

This concept is accepted in contemporary medical ethics and law.[3] In this chapter we appeal to the concept of physicians as fiduciaries of patients based on the work of Dr. John Gregory[4,5] and of health care organizations as fiduciaries of patients based on the work of Dr. Thomas Percival[6] as a core concept for the ethics of physician leadership in contemporary medicine.

We begin by identifying two professional virtues, diffidence and compassion, as vital to the fulfillment of fiduciary responsibility to patients. We then deploy these virtues in preventive ethics strategies for dealing with two major problems in physician-health care-organization interactions, what we call strategic procrastination (e.g., physicians delaying implementation of practice guidelines or organizational managers responding slowly to urgent problems) and strategic ambiguity (e.g., physicians exaggerating symptoms to justify inapplicability of practice guidelines or organizational managers making financial promises without articulating a dollar amount or timeline for delivery).

We propose that physician leaders should adopt a preventive ethics response to both strategic procrastination and strategic ambiguity by pointing them out when they occur and emphasizing that they compromise co-fiduciary responsibility. In addition, to prevent strategic procrastination, physician leaders should serve as role models of accountability by changing organizational policy and practice in a timely manner when intellectually obligated to do so. To prevent strategic ambiguity, physician leaders should become role models of transparency by being explicit in their communications.[1]

The Current Ethical Climate in Health Care Organizations

In today's climate of fiscal constraint, the relationship between physician leaders and health care organizations is often characterized by tension and even open conflict, rather than by routine cooperation. This tension can especially manifest itself in the current relationship between physicians and managed care organizations (MCOs).[7] Indeed, MCOs act as if, they do not or even deny, that they have fiduciary responsibility to patients; that responsibility rests with physicians. In such organizational cultures, physicians and organizations can have sharply divergent interests. In contrast, hospitals usually acknowledge their commitment to fiduciary responsibility to patient care, in conjunction with physicians. In our judgment, the tension between physician leaders and organizational managers, when it occurs, owes more to divergent interests than to lack of shared responsibility.

The Concept of Co-Fiduciary Responsibility for Patients

Physicians as Fiduciaries of Patients

The ethical concept of the physician as a fiduciary of the patient means that the physician is:

- An authority, i.e., possesses expert knowledge and skills about how to protect and promote the health-related interests of the patient.
- Committed to using that expertise primarily for the benefit of the patient and to making self-interest a systematically secondary condition.[3,8]

This concept comes to us from the history of medical ethics during the late eighteenth and early nineteenth centuries. One of the earliest and philosophically most sophisticated accounts in modern medical ethics of the concept of the physician as a fiduciary was developed by Dr. John Gregory (1724-1773) of Scotland. Gregory developed this concept on the basis of the philosophy of science and medicine of Francis Bacon (1561-1626) and the philosophical ethics of his contemporary, David Hume (1711-1776). Gregory wrote his medical ethics largely in response to the entrepreneurial, self-interested practice of medicine of the time. Gregory was very concerned that unbridled self-interest of physicians led to bias and prejudice, thus undermining the scientific quality of clinical judgment and practice. This intellectual failure had ethically significant consequences, namely, imperiling the health and lives of patients.[4,5]

Gregory proposed important and still-timely responses to these ethical challenges. He began his critique by noting that medicine needed to become more rigorously scientific than it was at the time. For Gregory, this meant that physician leaders should apply Baconian scientific methods to medical education, clinical practice, and research. To achieve this goal, physicians must cultivate the capacity of being "open to conviction." For Gregory, being "open to conviction" meant that physicians should base clinical judgment and practice on solid scientific grounds and be willing to change their thinking and practice on the basis of evidence. Physicians should, therefore, cultivate the professional intellectual virtue of diffidence, i.e., a studied indifference to current medical theories and practices. This studied indifference means that scientifically based criticism of theory and practice and the willingness to change on the basis of evidence become routine, just as evidence-based medicine now teaches. Gregory argued, correctly, that practicing medicine according to the virtue of diffidence would result in medical practice that conforms to standards of intellectual excellence. David Mechanic's recent and powerful call for an "evidence-based culture" of medicine makes Gregory's point in more contemporary terms.[9] Evidence-based, scientifically disciplined thinking counts now as diffidence, the first component of the concept of the physician as fiduciary.

Gregory appealed to Hume's ethics as the basis for the second component of the physician as fiduciary. According to Hume's ethics, we all have the capacity for sympathy, and this basic human capacity helps to generate the moral virtue of compassion, i.e., recognizing when others are in pain, distress, or suffering and seeking routinely and promptly to help them. As a result of developing the virtue of compassion and living by its requirements, we become the sort of people for whom the interests of others become our primary concern and for whom self-interest becomes a systematically secondary concern.[4,5] The emphasis on the virtue of compassion continues in contemporary medical ethics,[10] as a does a concern for empathy.[11]

Cultivating diffidence and compassion helps to make the physician's life of service to science and to patients routine. Acting primarily on self-interest by neglecting either diffidence or compassion undermines this life of service to others and therefore becomes the principal source of poor patient care. Gregory viewed vanity and other forms of self-interest as the altar on which many thousands of patient's lives have been sacrificed. Gregory thought that the moral catastrophe of unbridled self-interest should be obvious to the physicians of his day, just as we should two centuries later.

Gregory's views can be readily updated to our time. Diffidence should now be understood to mean that evidence-based medicine should govern clinical judgment and practice to the greatest extent possible.[9,12] Physicians should routinely and without objection accept accountability for processes and outcomes of care when they are measured against scientifically reliable standards. This contemporary version of diffidence will reduce uncontrolled clinical variation and therefore help optimize patients' health and functional status. Compassion has a timeless dimension, making Gregory's advice on this virtue directly relevant today. Physicians should, without prompting, respond promptly to and seek to relieve and prevent the pain, distress, and suffering of their patients.

Health Care Organizations as Fiduciaries of Patients

The next generation of English-language medical ethics after Gregory accepted the concept of fiduciary responsibility of hospitals. The English physician-ethicist, Thomas Percival (1740-1803) wrote his medical ethics in response to disputes among physicians, surgeons, and apothecaries that had paralyzed operations of the Manchester infirmary, to the detriment of patients. Percival proposed a series of procedures for physician cooperation that were intended to curb self-interest and focus physicians' main concern on the well-being of hospitalized patients. One of the procedures required that hospitals create "registers" to record the processes and outcomes of care, what we now call databases. Sharing these data with physicians and surgeons would enable them to improve their hospital care and, by comparing their hospital practice to their office practice, their outpatient care. To facilitate improvement of patient care, Percival proposed that hospitals hold monthly meetings to share data and encourage improvements in patient care.[6]

Percival addressed the then controversial topic of rationing of scarce resources. Resource use, he argued in a prescient fashion, should not be evaluated on the basis of the cost-per-encounter but rather on overall cost. Thus, when a single dose of a more expensive drug is more effective and less expensive than the cumulative cost of cheaper alternatives, the more expensive drug should be used. Moreover, when patients' lives can be saved, cost is irrelevant. By implication, strict control of resources is permitted when disease is self-limiting and choosing the least expensive alternative would not alter the outcome.[6] Current practices of evidence-based drug substitution to manage soaring formulary costs extend this line of reasoning into contemporary health care management.

Physicians & Health Care Organizations as Co-Fiduciaries of Patients

We can interpret these and the other management strategies that Percival proposed as designed to create an organizational culture of fiduciary professionalism. In such an organizational culture, physicians and health care organizations would adopt the concept of co-fiduciary responsibility for patients. Physicians would conform their clinical judgment and practice to the virtues of diffidence and compassion. Organizational managers would create and fund practices and procedures that support physicians' professional virtues.

Percival was aware that his proposals might be expensive. In response, he expressed complete confidence that hospitals with a culture of "purist beneficence...can never want contributions adequate to their liberal support."[6] Since the 1980s in the United States, with the introduction of Medicare's prospective payment system followed by the cost control of MCOs in the 1990s and ever-tighter Medicare and Medicaid budgets, contemporary health care organizations do want for their support and have given up all expectations for something as extravagant as liberal support. As a consequence, physician leaders who expect to survive today's environment would be irrational and irresponsible not to make fiscal health a priority. However, if the emphasis on fiscal health overwhelms co-fiduciary obligations of physicians and health care organizations, we will have regressed to the world of the primacy of self-interest, which Gregory and Percival would rightly have us see as moral anathema for patients, physicians, and health care organizations alike.

Preventive Ethics Strategies for Sustaining an Organizational Culture of Co-Fiduciary Responsibility

We can now apply the Gregory's and Percival's concept of the co-fiduciary responsibility of physicians and health care organizations in the form of preventive ethics strategies for keeping individual and organizational interests in their proper places and therefore sustaining and strengthening an organizational culture of fiduciary professionalism. Following Gregory and Percival, we propose new preventive ethics strategies—first to promote diffidence and then to promote compassion in the contemporary medical leadership of health care organizations.[1]

Preventive Ethics Strategies to Promote Diffidence

Preventive ethics strategies to promote diffidence start with shared commitment between physicians and health care organizations for excellence in patient care. To implement this strategy, physicians must be committed to evidence-based medicine, even if this means changing one's or one's group's longstanding practices. Health care organizations must commit the resources needed to implement best practices, e.g., by providing the necessary support for information technology.

Preventive ethics to promote diffidence should make what we call strategic procrastination a primary focus of concern. Physicians employ this tactic when they don't cooperate with data collection, when they don't attend quality assurance meetings, when they delay implementation of practice guidelines, or when they claim to be an exception to guidelines because so many of their patients have greater acuity. The goal of such strategic procrastination appears to be preservation of physician autonomy and power to continue old practices undisturbed.

Health care organizations employ strategic procrastination when leaders and managers delay funding of data collection, management, analysis, or dissemination. In addition, health care organizations can respond very slowly to problems with data systems. The goal of strategic procrastination appears to be to withhold and redeploy capital and, perhaps, to retain power.

The first preventive ethics strategy in response to strategic procrastination should be for physician leaders to expose this practice as obstructing co-fiduciary responsibility. In addition, physician leaders, after soliciting the support of senior hospital managers, should serve as role models of accountability and willingness to change one's practice when intellectually obliged to do so. Physician leaders should especially be role models of accountability to non-physician colleagues—e.g., to nurses and social workers regarding improvement of discharge planning, to pharmacologists regarding prevention of drug-drug interaction, and to financial officers on the costs of components of processes of care. Health care organizations should commit needed resources and physician leaders should solicit their colleagues' input on how these resource allocations can best promote co-fiduciary responsibility. Failure to create such involvement not only prevents physician "buy-in" but also encourages physicians to procrastinate even more. Physician leaders should also advocate with trustees and senior leadership for these preventive ethics strategies as being essential to an organizational culture of diffidence and, therefore, professionalism.

Preventive Ethics Strategies to Promote Compassion

Preventive ethics strategies to promote compassion also start with shared commitment to excellence in patient care. Compassion, as an essential component of excellent patient care, requires physicians not to cause unnecessary stress and anxiety in their patients. Physician leaders should treat their professional colleagues with a decent minimum of compassion, modeled on the compassion with which physicians are expected to treat patients.

Preventive ethics intended to promote compassion should make what we call strategic ambiguity its primary focus of concern. Strategic ambiguity in communication from organizational leadership leads to uncertainty, confusion, and, even worse, distrust on the part of physicians. Physicians employ strategic ambiguity at the bedside when they exaggerate symptoms to justify the inapplicability of practice guidelines, when they decline to provide evidence that many of their patients are sicker, when they claim to be providing excellent patient care but are unable or unwilling to articulate the standards they used to reach that judgment, and when they make vague, unsubstantiated criticism of organizational leadership. The goal of these tactics appears to be preservation of power that might be lost if they met conditions of transparency. Another goal appears to be avoidance of the hard work of institutional improvement and reform.

Organizational leadership employs the tactics of strategic ambiguity when it makes financial promises without articulating a timetable or dollar amount, when it emphasizes quality without a plan of implementation, when it orders a subordinate to terminate an employee but then expresses perplexity to the employee as to why termination happened, and when it invokes or expresses support for excellence without a detailed account of what it means by excellence. The goal of these tactics also appears to be preservation of power and avoidance of accountability that might be lost if leadership met conditions of transparency.

The first preventive ethics strategy for physician leaders to employ should be to promptly point out strategic ambiguity when it occurs and to request, even insist if necessary, that conditions of transparency be satisfied. Physician leaders should be role models of transparency by being precise in their patient records, by providing evidence of variation of acuity, and by leading efforts to improve and reform organizations. Organizational leadership should be explicit in communications, justify decisions, and own up to and stand behind decisions, especially when they are controversial or have unexpected consequences.

Physicians and health care organizations should hold each other mutually accountable for creating and sustaining an organizational culture of mutual trust. Physician leaders should advocate for evaluation of senior leadership, including themselves, by trustees and corporate officers on this basis.

Sometimes, strategic procrastination and strategic ambiguity can become synergistic, with procrastination undermining compassion and ambiguity undermining diffidence. Strategic procrastination in the development of best practices puts patients at risk for inadequate clinical management, which can result in unnecessary pain, distress, and suffering. Strategic ambiguity becomes anathema to the transparency required by evidence-based medicine. The preventive ethics strategies proposed above, in our judgment, have the advantage of preventing this unfortunate synergy and the organizational culture of cynicism that such synergy promotes. Physician leaders should be especially attentive to the emergence of such cynicism as symptomatic of an organizational culture that has drifted very far indeed from the requirements of co-fiduciary responsibility.

Conclusion

Gregory understood that fulfilling fiduciary responsibility requires individual integrity, i.e., sustained commitment of each physician to practice medicine according to standards of intellectual and moral excellence, as required by diffidence and compassion. Percival added to Gregory's medical ethics the crucial insight that maintenance of individual professional integrity requires a supportive organizational culture. Today, physician leaders and, as a consequence, the health care organizations for which they are responsible may be at unrecognized risk of losing Percival's insight. It is as if fiduciary responsibility of physicians and health care organizations exist, but on parallel lines that never meet.

To be sure, parallel responsibility is better than denial of responsibility, which often can, unfortunately, define organizational culture. However, parallel responsibility results at best in an anemic organizational culture, in which the tactics of strategic procrastination and strategic ambiguity can flourish. The ethical and leadership antidote, which we take from Gregory and Percival, is for physician leaders to create and sustain an organizational culture based on the reality, not the rhetoric, of shared fiduciary responsibility for patients. Mechanic calls for a new professionalism.[9] Perhaps it is more accurate to say that we need to recover and re-invigorate the concept of shared fiduciary responsibility that we inherit from two giants in the history of medical ethics, Gregory and Percival.

References

1. Chervenak, F., and McCullough, L. "Physicians and Hospitals as Co-fiduciaries of Patients: Rhetoric or Reality?" *Journal of Healthcare Management*, 48(3):172-9, May-June 2003.

2. McCullough, L. "A Basic Concept in the Clinical Ethics of Managed Care: Physicians and Institutions as Economically Disciplined Moral Co-Fiduciaries of Populations of Patients." *Journal of Medical Philosophy* 24(1):77-97, Feb. 1999.

3. McCullough, L., and Chervenak, F. *Ethics in Obstetrics and Gynecology*. New York, N.Y.: Oxford University Press, 1994.

4.   McCullough, L. *John Gregory (1724-1773) and the Invention of Professional Medical Ethics and the Profession of Medicine.* Dordrecht, Netherlands: Kluwer Academic Publishers, 1998.

5.   McCullough, L., Ed. *John Gregory's Writing on Medical Ethics and Philosophy of Medicine.* Dordrecht, Netherlands: Kluwer Academic Publishers, 1998.

6.   Percival, T. *Medical Ethics, or a Code of Institutes and Precepts Adapted to the Professional Conduct of Physicians and Surgeons.* London: Russell and Johnson, 1803.

7.   Chervenak, F., and McCullough, L. "Responding to the Ethical Challenges Posed by the Business Tools of Managed Care in the Practice of Obstetrics and Gynecology." *American Journal of Obstetrics and Gynecology* 173(3 Pt 1):523-7, Sept. 1996.

8.   Chervenak, F., and McCullough, L. "The Moral Foundation of Medical Leadership: The Professional Virtues of the Physician as Fiduciary of the Patient." *American Journal of Obstetrics and Gynecology* 184(5):875-80, April 2001.

9.   Mechanic, D. "Managed Care and the Imperative for a New Professional Ethic." *Health Affairs* 19(5):100-11, Sept.-Oct. 2000.

10. Pellegrino, E., and Thomasma, D. *The Virtues in Medical Practice.* New York, N.Y.: Oxford University Press, 1993.

11. Spiro, H, and others. *Empathy and the Practice of Medicine.* New Haven, Conn.: Yale University Press, 1993.

12. Evidence-Based Medicine Working Group. "Evidence-Based Medicine: A New Approach to Teaching the Practice of Medicine." *JAMA* 268(17):2420-5, Nov. 4, 1992.

Frank Chervenak, MD, MMM, CPE, FACPE is Chair of the Obstetrics and Gynecology Department at New York Weill Cornell Medical Center in New York City.

Laurence McCullough, PhD is Professor of Medicine at Baylor College of Medicine Center for Ethics in Houston, Texas.

Chapter 13

Communicating in a Changed World

by Barbara J. Linney, MA

The climate in a health care organization has always been stressful because life and death crises happen there. People are even more on edge these days because of shrinking resources, nurse shortages, the threat of malpractice suits, and increased patient demands. One way to cope and lessen the stress is to communicate calmly and clearly with co-workers and patients.

The main skills needed for good communication are talking so that people will want to listen to you, listening so that people will want to talk to you, and writing so that people will want to read what you have written.

There are ways to improve these skills and enable communication to take place. If someone absolutely does not want to communicate with you, nothing will work. It takes two people putting forth energy for a good interaction to happen, but if you will work on your techniques, you will find more people will respond to you in a positive way.

Talking

What will make people listen to you when you talk?

- Pronounce your words clearly. Enunciate. Don't mumble. You need to use energy to project your voice to the other person. He or she should not have to strain to hear you. It is very annoying to try to have a conversation with someone you cannot hear. However, the opposite, yelling, is also unacceptable. Some will yell back at you, increase the hostility, and create anxiety for all who are watching. Others will shrink away in fear but plot ways to get even with you later.

- Don't talk too quickly or too slowly. Southerners sometimes have to speed up. Northerners sometimes have to slow down. Midwesterners usually have it about right.

- Look at the other person. Look as if you are enjoying the conversation. You don't have to stare the person down, but if your eyes wander all over the room or you always look over their shoulders, listeners have a hard time paying attention to what you are saying. They secretly speculate about what you are looking at rather than listening to what you are saying.

- Eliminate the word "just." I have been in meetings in which everyone started his or her report with, "I just want to update you on...." Sometimes they were describing the biggest event of the year. Adding the word "just" implies that what you are about to say is not important. If you leave it out, the message is more powerful.

- Use average size words. If you sling around a lot of jargon or large words that most people do not know, you alienate them. Patients do not always know what MRI or myocardial infarction means.

- Don't talk longer than a couple of minutes without letting the other person talk. Taking turns was a valuable thing to learn when we were young and we never outgrow the need to do it. "Most people fade fast and lose interest if they don't feel like an equal partner in a conversation. Talking too much is like weighing down a seesaw so that you cannot bob up and down with your playmate. It takes all the fun out of the activity."[1]

According to Jung's concept of extravert and introvert, extraverts talk and then figure out what they think; introverts figure out what they think and then talk. The introverts have valuable information if you give them time to say it. It's the job of any physician executive to be sure he or she gets ideas from both kinds. Otherwise, unneeded resentment builds in the organization. It requires restraining the quick talkers some and encouraging those who do not speak up quickly.

- Be willing to tell what you feel about a subject as well as what you think. Give a personal example. "I think we would have better meetings with the doctors if we met at 6 p.m. instead of 9 p.m. Frankly, I'm just too tired to concentrate at 9 p.m. after I've worked a 12-hour shift."

- Avoid teasing. People fear others will humiliate them for the way they look, for what they say, or for what they have done. They cope with this fear in several ways. Some try to talk a lot and thus control the words. If they are doing the talking, they may not be hurt by someone else's words. Others do not speak up for fear of saying something wrong. The very witty and those able to come back with a quick retort are usually the only ones who enjoy teasing.

Teasing can be fun between equals, but often it is a secret form of aggression, and it strips its victim of power unless both parties are equally good at the quick barb. Teasing usually allows the one doing the teasing to feel "one up." This occasionally feels good, but it eliminates closeness and builds resentment. A doctor teasing nurses is not good unless the nurses feel equally free to tease the doctor. The latter is rare. If you tease your children a lot, you may want to rethink that. You are not equals. The child usually feels very bad, even though he or she may be laughing.

Avoid telling jokes unless you are positive no one would be offended. Laws on sexual harassment are enforced more every year. Unless the joke's on you, you are wise to leave it out.

- Don't overuse big emotions, such as anger or tears. There are times when we are angry and the other person must know it, but those times are rare. It's similar to the little boy who hollered "wolf." If you are angry in most of your exchanges, people will learn to tune you out or will automatically scream back at you. If you cry often at work, people will not listen to you or take you seriously.

Big emotions usually interfere with communication. The listener is often threatened, frightened, or repulsed by a show of uncontrolled emotion, and he or she cannot hear the words being spoken. The person raging or crying also cannot hear when the listener responds.

What can you do when emotions are raging?

When you are the speaker, "Writing in a journal about people or situations that have evoked in us anger, anxiety, or a sense of defeat helps to stabilize our psychological situation and strengthen our ego. It helps us to 'get a handle' on our emotions without repressing them, and to get a look at the giant that threatens to swallow us. If we do this before we get into a discussion that might become highly emotional, the chances are good that we can express our feelings to the other person and not be consumed by them."[2]

When you are the listener, if you are feeling strong and collected, it is helpful if you can let the emotional person vent for a few moments. You might then respond, "I can see that you are angry, and I'm not surprised. What can I do to help?" If you are not up to being in the presence of so much negative energy, you might say, "I'll be glad to talk about this when you are calmer."

- Know what you want. It is a good idea to prepare for important conversations. By writing ahead of time, you can clearly focus on what you want and on what price you are willing to pay to get it. The following questions can help you think through an important interaction ahead of time. It is not cheating to prepare; it is wise.

What do you think about the situation?

What do you feel about the situation?

What do you want?

What will be the good or the bad consequences if you get it?

What are you willing to do to get what you want?

What do you think the other person wants?

Can you give any of what he or she wants?

The following is an example of using these questions. I was in the middle of a business interaction between two friends of mine. They did not know each other. Bill wanted Joe to put on a program for a group he was in. Bill was outraged at the price Joe asked and wanted me to pass a nasty message back to Joe.

What do you think about the situation? I think Bill got angry when I would not do something he asked me to do. I would not call Joe and tell him that instead of Bill's paying him to speak, Joe would have to pay Bill's group thousands of dollars for it to even let him speak there.

What do you feel about the situation? At first I felt angry. Now I feel hurt by the rejection. Bill has not talked to me for three months.

What do you want? To have lunch together occasionally, to talk, and to share ideas but not to have him start trying to tell me outlandish things to do again.

What will be the good or the bad consequences if you get what you want? Good—I'd have his stimulating, mind-spurring thoughts in me again. Bad—He'd get into the bossiness again, or I'd get tired of laughing at his jokes, if we had too much contact. (I laughed whether they were funny or not because most of the time I got enough good out of the interactions to make it worth it.)

What are you willing to do to get what you want? Call him and say, "Could we have lunch and talk about why we don't talk anymore?"

What do you think the other person wants? To be one up. Maybe an apology. I'm not sure what he wants—that's what I could find out if we talked.

Can you give him any of what he wants? I can apologize and say I didn't handle the situation well, but I can't be in a friendship where he slips into giving me orders.

- Use good body language. How you say something and how you look when you say it are as important as what you say. What causes someone to understand you and respond well to you? "In a famous 1971 study, psychologist Albert Mehrabian found that 7 percent of understanding depends on the words you use, 38 percent depends on your tone of voice, and 55 percent depends on your nonverbal body language."[3]

Facial expression and voice communicate much more than you realize. A listener understands and interprets your message more through the tone of your voice and the look of your body than through your words. "No, I'm not angry!" said harshly conveys the message that you are angry. "I really love that!" said sarcastically implies that you don't like it at all. People complain about getting mixed signals when words, tone of voice, and body language send different messages. They will believe the tone of your voice and the look on your face much more than the words you say.

Alexander claims people have a hard time accepting these facts. "The reality is that few people accept responsibility for anything more than their words. They have never learned that a harsh tone can deny the gentlest of words...."[4] Most people refuse to believe it if they are the ones doing the talking, but they quickly believe it if someone else is doing the talking.

A positive voice is cheerful, satisfied, concerned, warm. A negative voice is sarcastic, scared, depressed, clipped, tense, too loud or soft. A positive face has a smile, an occasional head nod, and eye contact. A negative face has a frown, smirk, or boring glare. A positive body is relaxed, leaning forward some, with open arms. Negative body language is pointing, wandering eyes, picking at your body.[5]

Be even more careful about your tone of voice when you talk on the telephone. We are often thrown into someone's voice mail unexpectedly if his or her line is busy. Do not leave a stumbling, mumbling message. If you are not prepared, hang up, write out what you want to say and call back. Recruiters and others will make judgments about whether or not you can do a management job by the quality of your voice and the coherence of your message on the phone.

Listening

Listening is the most important ingredient in establishing rapport with people. "Relationships are established best through one-to-one meetings of the key invested people, not through e-mails, phone calls, or faxes. Find constructive ways to meet with the people you wish to influence."[6]

You have work to do when you are listening. Most resources describe the process as active listening. You move your eyes and head some, you make some encouraging noises, and you let the speaker know you have understood the words, sentences, and overall meaning.

Active listening has gotten some bad press, because people have overused the term, "I hear what you are saying." Also, if someone is rampaging, and I say, "You seem to be angry," a natural response might be, "You're damned right I'm angry." Active listening is a good technique, but how and when you use it needs to vary if you do not want to further alienate the person you are talking to.

"Active listening involves a restatement of either the message or the feeling of the speaker without giving advice, analyzing, or probing."[7] It is the place to begin when listening to someone with a problem. But you do not want to overdo active listening either, because the speaker may feel that you are acting like a parrot or a robot also do not quickly interrupt and say, "I know how you feel," or give advice.

Listening is an art that starts with attentive silence. When my daughter was young, if I did not look at her when she talked to me, she would say, "Turn your face, Mama." Shortly after she could talk, she knew I had to be looking at her to really be paying attention. Adults know this, too, whether they tell you or not. It's your job to hold your eyes and body so that others know you are paying attention.

Young children talk a lot, so when I couldn't listen anymore, I said so and told them I would listen more later. We need to deal with adults in the same way. If you cannot pay attention, say, "I'm swamped with this project right now, but I can give you my undivided attention at 3 p.m. Could you come back then?" Then be sure to give them the time at 3 p.m.

Try not to make a habit of pretending to listen when you are not. People will come to distrust you. However, all of us have been in long meetings when listening simply was not in us anymore. At that point, pretending to listen is better than throwing your arms back with a deep sigh or closing your eyes in a bored slouch. Such behavior has a negative effect on those who may still be paying attention.

Listening is hard work. "While an average speech rate for many people is about 200 words per minute, most of us can think about four times that speed. With all that extra think time, the ineffective listener lets his mind wander. His brain takes excursions to review the events of yesterday, or plan tomorrow, or solve a business problem...or sleep."[8] You have to work to control your mind and make it concentrate on what is being said. If you are troubled by an impending malpractice suit, a divorce, or a child who is having problems, your capacity to listen will diminish drastically. You will need to be patient with yourself in those circumstances and perhaps say to the person speaking, "I am a bit distracted. Can you tell me that again?"

If you decide you are willing to expend the energy to listen, here are some techniques that will help you listen so people will want to talk to you:

- Be quiet. You cannot be listening if you are talking or you are thinking hard about what you are going to say next. If you get very anxious about not knowing what to say when they finish, try putting all your energy into listening and then tell them, "I need to think about this. Can I get back with you in a while to talk more?" Often "conversation in the U.S. is a competitive exercise in which the first person to draw a breath is declared the listener."[9] If you're guilty of this, don't continue it.

- Use your body to let the person know you are there. Look at him or her. Don't let your eyes wander all over the room. Sit attentively but not tensely, not slouching or lying down. None of these are good positions for listening: lying on the sofa watching television, reading the paper, opening your regular mail or glancing at your computer screen when an e-mail pops up.

- Give an occasional "uh huh" or nod to let people know you are following their train of thought. If you are not, ask them a question before you let them go on for too long and you are really lost. Don't overdo head nodding. It can look as if you are agreeing with everything the person is saying. Don't over do the "uh huh"s. I knew someone who did that constantly. Every sound she made sounded like "Shut up, shut up, shut up" so I can have my turn to talk.

- Ask nonjudgmental questions. "Can you say a little more? I'm not sure I understand. Will you try me again?" Don't ask, "Why on earth did you do that?" There is absolutely no decent answer to that question, and the person doing the asking is implying, "You are an idiot!" You may be right, but if you want communication to continue, you will have to discipline yourself not to say everything you think. "Why" almost always indicates negative judgment.

- Restate some of what the person has said. "Let me see if I understand. You think Dr. X is showing up for his emergency department shift with alcohol on his breath."

- Make a guess about a feeling you think the person is having if it seems appropriate. "I can see why that would make you sad." They may reply, "I'm not sad, I'm angry." It doesn't matter that you are wrong. They will correct you, and you have gotten to a deeper level of communication when you find out how someone feels about a subject. The person will experience a sense of relief and sometimes release when he or she identifies the feeling.

It is not easy to listen. We would all rather be the center of attention, doing all the talking. This is not a bad fact, just a fact. But if we do not learn to take turns, if we do not learn to listen, we will not have a chance of being heard.

"One big clue that we are not really focused on what someone is saying is how quickly we respond after he has finished speaking. When a person is talking, it doesn't mean we use that time to figure out what to say next. It's just the opposite; we use that time to listen. Then by waiting a few beats after that person is finished, especially when the subject matter is complex or highly charged, we give ourselves an extra moment to compose our thoughts and respond with a higher degree of sensitivity."[10]

Conflict

Many people would claim they behave in ways that make interpersonal communication go more smoothly, but they also might admit that, when situations get hostile, they forget everything and often react in ways that they don't like. Confrontation is difficult. People usually deal with it in one of two ways. They verbally attack, using the energy of anger to spur them on, or they withdraw, say nothing, and often plot revenge.

Confronting someone in a calm, firm voice takes courage. I'd like to suggest a how-to process that can help you control yourself if you tend to explode and help you get the nerve to confront if you tend to withdraw. I mentioned earlier that it is helpful to prepare for important conversations. That is especially true if you are in a heated situation. Try filling in the blanks in this short formula:

When you (do so and so),

I feel (or react in this way),

Because (I think something).

I'd like you to (do so and so).

Examples:

When you verbally attack me and defend your position when I ask you to do something, I get angry and I avoid telling you what you need to hear, because I think nothing will be accomplished and I dread your reaction. Next time, I'd like you to listen until I finish and think about it, and then we can discuss it.

When you come to me with every emergency department problem you have, I feel angry, because I can only deal with one dying person at a time. I'd like you to make some of the decisions yourself. I trust your judgment.

Sometimes you take the process a step further and tell what the consequences will be if behavior is not changed.

When you leave your charts unreviewed for two weeks, the rest of the staff and I are frustrated (angry), because we can't properly take care of patients and get our work done. I want you to complete them in three days. If not, I'll alert the medical records committee.

Using the formula, continue to write to find out exactly what you want to say. When you actually speak to the person, the formula will take a slightly different form. The following is what I might actually tell the person concerning the first example:

Sometimes I need to ask you to change a behavior. When I do, you quickly defend your position and verbally attack me. As a result, I dread telling you something. I put it off, and yet I know you are going to suffer in your performance evaluation if you do not change. In the future, when I have something difficult to tell you, I'm going to say, "I have something difficult to tell you." I'd like you to listen until I finish and think about it, and then we can get together to discuss it.

When you get ready to talk to the person, you may not tell them exactly what you have written, but the formula can help you get clear about what aggravates you, what part you play in creating the problem, and what it is you want to happen. If you get angry, you can cuss and vent and scream on paper and then throw it away. When you spill those feelings on people, they are usually either so angry themselves or so frightened that they cannot hear what it is you want them to do.

If you are the one who often withdraws from conflict, you can sometimes get the courage to speak up, because you have written out exactly what you plan to say. You don't have to have the notes with you. Your brain has thought them and seen them on paper so it will usually remember them. You can also practice saying the words out loud so that your brain will have also heard them.

Some things you discover when you are writing you will not want to tell. For example, that you are frightened about something. To say that may make you seem too vulnerable. Someone might say, "She's not tough enough to do this job. Let's get rid of her." So you don't always tell what you feel, but it is very important for you to know what you feel. When you don't know your feelings, you can continue to act in unproductive ways (e.g., as an angry or frightened little boy or girl) and wonder why life and your job are not good. When you are aware of what you feel, you can move through it and feel something that is often better than the first impression. When you know your feelings, you can remind yourself that you are grown, that you have options, that this person does not have your very life in his or her hands.

If writing seems too disagreeable a task, try telling all of this to a friend before you talk to the one who has annoyed you, but don't leave it there. If the information never gets back to the person who caused you the trouble, there is no chance for the situation to improve.

When someone irritates us, we want to complain to a friend because it feels good to do so. We want to vent. I do not think this human behavior will stop, but if the listener could let the talker vent for a while and then encourage him or her to prepare to talk to the offending person, office gossip would sometimes have a productive end rather than just fueling the "poor-me" fire.

Writing

In the area of communication, there will probably come a time when you have to write. What will make people want to read what you have written?

- Make it short. We may or may not be getting lazier, with shorter attention spans as some sources claim, but we are all definitely busy. Even the brightest executives want documents to be short, because they need to get through them in a hurry.

- Have enough "white space"—areas on a page where there are no words. Do you remember when, in the seventh grade, you started to read that larger geography book with more words on a page? You struggled through two columns of heavy words and then turned the page to find a picture that took up half the page. Weren't you happy, relieved? When we grow up, we pretend that we get over that thrill, but we don't. None of us want to look at a page that is heavy and mostly black with words. If there are good top, bottom, and side margins, with spaces between paragraphs and perhaps a list in the middle with more white space around it, we are invited to read what is on the page rather than repelled by it.

- Avoid needless repetition. Do not repeat the same word many times. The reader begins to hear the singsong repetition of the word rather than your message. It is fine to repeat the same word when you are first generating your thoughts, but you need to cut them later.

Writing needs to be a two-part process. First, you come up with ideas without criticizing them at all. If you judge every word as you go, the creative part of you will get tired and will stop sending messages. Just write down or dictate the words as they come to you. Become very critical when you edit. Circle all the repeated words and try to eliminate most of them, unless you are repeating the word to emphasize its importance or changing the word would confuse the reader.

- Don't be verbose. Don't write the same idea a second time using different words: end result, final conclusion, personal opinion, unexpected surprise. Always use fewer words rather than more. "In the event that" can simply be "if." "In view of the fact that" can be "Because."[11] Elbow says, "Every word omitted keeps another reader with you."[12] It is especially important for physicians to use simple words and phrases whenever they can because so often they must use the long technical words of their profession. Too many words of three or more syllables make for heavy reading. Resist using complicated medical terminology unless you are communicating with your medical colleagues.

- Use nonsexist language. Avoid words that imply only a man or a woman could do the job. Instead of businessman, write business executive, manager, or business person. Instead of chairman say chair or chairperson. When writing to a woman, use the title "Ms." unless you know she would prefer "Mrs." or "Miss." "Mr." indicates the person you are addressing is a man but explains nothing about his marital status. "Ms." does the same for a woman.

  Instead of using the masculine pronoun (he, his, him) when referring to a group that includes both men and women, make the subject of the sentence plural and thus neutral. Example: Employees must submit their travel expenses by Monday. Sometimes you will have to use the singular pronoun. When you do, write "he or she" or "he/she." Too many of these expressions will sound awkward, but it is no longer acceptable to use just "he."

- Always choose precise words rather than vague words. Instead of "nice house" say "brick house." Instead of "circumstance" put "Hurricane Floyd." Use strong verbs rather than ones hidden in many words. "Decide" is stronger than "make a decision." "Buy" is better than "make a purchase." "Help" is clearer than "give assistance."

- Don't use jargon unless you are absolutely sure the listener understands it. Jargon, in its broadest definition, is any language that is hard to understand. Sometimes it acts as a shield for those who don't have much to say. It can be specialized vocabulary that a particular group of people understands. Teenagers find a different set of words every two or three years that, they hope, will confuse their parents.

  Accountants, chemists, bankers, doctors, and others have special terms that must be defined when they are working with the general public. Abbreviations that the listener does not understand are jargon. It's the writer's job to find out what the reader knows and doesn't know. When it comes to abbreviations, if you are in doubt, write it out.

In academic institutions a particular style or jargon is often necessary to pass muster in certain classes, but be careful to reassess its use if you are writing for a non-academic audience.

Often jargon is phony, inflated, and uselessly complex language. A client told me once, "If I speak and write so others understand me, they will steal my job." The opposite is more often true—jargon interferes with communication and could cause you to lose your job. People get angry if you use difficult words without explaining their meaning. They put your memos in the trash and do not do what you have asked them to do.

- Avoid trite phrases. Overworked expressions make a reader switch from paying attention to your message to being irritated that you are saying the same old thing. "The bottom line," "the whole nine yards," "I need your input," and "paradigm" are terms that need a few years' rest. "Coaching" and "leverage" are close to being overworked. If you can finish the following statements, they have probably been overused.

  Enclosed

  We're sorry for any

  It has come to our

  Please call at your earliest

  If you have additional questions, feel

  Try substituting new words. Examples for the first and second phrases might be, "Here is the information you asked for in your letter of June 5," and "Thanks for your patience with this delay."[11]

- Tone or manner of expression is as evident in the written word as it is in the spoken word. Business correspondence used to have a stuffy, legalistic tone. Now companies like a conversational, friendly tone that sounds as if a person, not a machine, wrote the letter. Pretend the reader is standing beside you. If you wouldn't say "per your request" to his or her face, don't write it in the letter.

  Use a positive tone whenever possible. "Saying that someone is 'interested in details' conveys a more positive tone than saying the individual is a 'nitpicker.' The word economical is more positive than stingy or cheap."[13]

Electronic Mail and Voice Mail

E-mail is a quick and efficient way to communicate with people, and, in many offices, thankfully, it has completely replaced the inner-office memo. You can be more informal than we used to advise on hard-copy memos, but don't get so routinely lax that people make judgments about your ability to spell and use proper grammar. A few mistakes here and there are acceptable but if all your messages are riddled with them, people will draw negative conclusions about your intelligence and competence.

Do not use all capital letters just because it is easier than dealing with the shift key. All caps are equivalent to yelling at someone, and they are very tiring to read. All lower case is better than all caps.

Do not criticize or correct people on e-mail—do it in a one-on-one conversation. Never type in e-mail or even in your office word processing program anything that you would not want everyone to read. You could accidentally hit the wrong button and send the message to everyone on the mail system, and people who have even a minimal knowledge of computers can go in your files and read what you have there. Some have told me that computer experts can get to files you have deleted if they choose to.

How To Make Writing Easier

I've given you several do's and don'ts, but what if you hate the whole writing process. Is there anything that would make you dread it less? The answer is writing more, but in a different way. Write 10 minutes a day, five days a week, on any subject that pops into your head. Use a kind of paper and pen that you like or type it on a word processor if that's easier for you. (Whatever paper or instrument you decide to write on I'll now refer to as your journal). Don't worry about spelling, punctuation, grammar, or anything that some English teacher told you to worry about. There is just one catch—you must start writing and not stop until the time is up. If you can't think of anything to write, just write, "I can't think of anything. I can't think of anything. This is one of the dumbest things I've ever done," but keep writing. Ideas will pop into your head if you keep writing that simply will not occur to you if you just sit and think.

If you were going to run in a 10-kilometer race on the weekend, you would need to do some daily running to get ready. The same is true for writing. You need to grease the machinery of your hand and brain to make them readily give you words when you need to write something.

Journal Writing

Journal writing will not only make the writing process easier but also can enhance your verbal communication skills and benefit you in other ways.

It can help you **organize your day.** You probably already make a "to do" list. Expand it. Gripe—"month end report for Mr. Jones. I hate the way he makes red marks and gives it back to me to do again just to show he has the power to do that. Performance appraisal for Dr. Thomas. UR meeting—

they go on and on without making a decision." You will think of the items to do much quicker if you write comments about them as you go. When you finish the journal entry, circle the tasks that came up that need to be done that day and assign them numbers in order of importance.

Writing in a journal can help you **get rid of frustration.** Anger is a physical phenomenon. You feel it somewhere in your body—knotted stomach, clinched fist, stiff neck. You cannot always avoid getting angry, but you need to get it out of your system for good health, and you don't want to dump it on the wrong person. You can dump it in your journal. Peter Elbow says, "Garbage in your head will poison you. Garbage on paper can safely be put in the waste paper basket."[14]

Writing quickly without stopping **taps your right brain creativity.** Most of us judge our ideas quickly. As soon as they pop into our heads, we think, "That will never work. Someone will think that is stupid." If you continue to write, the censor who seems to sit on your shoulder is thwarted and cannot continue to judge every thought. Thus, the right brain will keep sending you fresh thoughts because you are receiving them and showing respect by writing them down. Some of the ideas will be useful, but not all. You have to get a fair number of ideas out to have a few that are good.

While writing, you can find **creative solutions to relationship problems.** If you and your boss or spouse or child disagree over the same topic repeatedly, write out the scene in your journal. Often you wish you had said something differently or had not cried or had not lost your temper. Write the scene the way you wish it had happened. Next time you'll be amazed at how the interaction is similar to what you wrote, because you stayed calm in your half of the conversation.

If you decide to write in a journal, keep it hidden or tear up any incriminating evidence. Writing will take you to places you didn't know you were going to go. If you momentarily hate your boss, it is helpful to write about it but harmful if anyone sees it. You do not have to keep what you write in order to benefit from having written it.

If you've recognized a communication skill you would like to improve, what activities will help you change?

- Practice on a friend.
- Practice in front of a video camera.
- Write about it in your journal.
- Put little reminder notes to yourself where no one else can see them—in your desk drawer or the medicine cabinet. Examples: I let others have a chance to talk. I am a good listener. I am a strong energetic speaker.

- Relax and talk to yourself. The brain is much like a computer. It can be programmed and reprogrammed. If you don't like what you are doing, start to talk to yourself about a positive change. Learn some kind of relaxation or meditation technique. Do the exercise every day for three weeks. Each time you finish doing the exercise, say a positive statement to yourself about some desired change. Examples: I control my temper. I speak up when I choose to. The subconscious is more receptive when your body is relaxed. After several weeks, you'll be aware that you are interacting with people differently.

Changing the way you communicate is not easy. It requires practicing new behavior that will feel awkward for a while, but the effort's worth it. "Nothing is more essential to success in any area of your life than the ability to communicate well. Nothing can compare to the joy of communicating love, of being heard and understood completely, of discovering some profound insight from another's mind, or of transmitting your own thoughts to a rapt audience."[15]

References

1. Stettner, M. *The Art of Winning Conversation.* Englewood Cliffs, N.J.: Prentice Hall, 1995, p. 82.

2. Sanford, J. *Between People, Communicating One-to-One.* New York, N.Y.: Paulist Press, 1982, p. 37.

3. Griffin, J. *How to Say It at Work.* Paramus, N.J.: Prentice Hall Press, 1998, p. 17.

4. Alexander, J. *Dare to Change.* New York, N.Y.: New American Library, 1984, p. 138.

5. Swets, P. *The Art of Talking So That People Will Listen.* Englewood Cliffs, N.J.: Prentice-Hall, 1983, p. 59.

6. Bellman, G. *Getting Things Done When You Are Not in Charge.* San Francisco, Calif.: Berrett-Koehler Publishers, Inc., 2001, p.51.

7. Carr, J. *Communicating and Relating.* Menlo Park, Calif.: Benjamin/ Cummings Publishing Co., Inc., 1979, p. 152.

8. Swets, P., *op. cit.,* p. 42.

9. Leech, T. *Say It like Shakespeare.* New York, N.Y.: McGraw-Hill, 2001, p 123.

10. Gilbert, M. *Communication Miracles at Work.* Berkeley, Calif.: Conari Press, 2002, p. 100.

11. Brill, L., and others. *How to Sharpen Your Business Writing Skills.* New York, N.Y.: American Management Association, 1985.

12. Elbow, P. *Writing Without Teachers.* London: Oxford University Press, 1973, p. 41.

13. Kolin, P. *Successful Writing at Work*. Lexington, Mass.: D.C. Heath and Co., 1980, p.13.

14. Elbow, P., *op. cit.*, p. 8.

15. Swets, P., *op. cit.*, p. 4.

Works Consulted but not Cited

Collins, S. *The Joy of Success, 10 Essential Skills for Getting the Success You Want*. New York, N.Y.: HarperCollins Publishers, 2003.

Goldberg, N. *Writing Down the Bones*. Boston, Mass.: Shambala, 1986.

Horton, S. *Thinking Through Writing*. Baltimore, Md.: Johns Hopkins University Press, 1982.

Klauser, H. *Writing on Both Sides of the Brain: Breakthrough Techniques for People Who Write*. San Francisco, Calif.: Harper and Row, Publishers, 1986.

Maltz, M. *Psycho-Cybernetics*. Hollywood, Calif.: Wilshire Book Co., 1960.

Milo, F. *How to Get Your Point Across in 30 Seconds—or Less*. New York, N.Y.: Simon and Schuster, 1986.

James, M., and Jongeward, D. *Born to Win*. Philippines: Addison-Wesley Publishing Co., Inc., 1971.

Website: www.hardatwork.com has a section called "Solve a problem." People write in about communication problems they are having at work and others respond with suggestions. Some of the hints are helpful—an example is how to deal with a co-worker who is full of resentment.

Barbara J. Linney, MA, is Vice President of Career Development for the American College of Physician Executives, Tampa, Florida.

Chapter 14

Making Conflict Work for You: Its Value, Sources, and Opportunities

by Edward J. O'Connor, PhD
and C. Marlena Fiol, PhD

After many months of continuous debate, administration has decided to move forward in implementing a new computerized OR scheduling system. You believe that it promises to streamline patient flow and lead to more efficient use of resources. However, resistance and conflict in your department regarding the new system appear to be growing.

Dr. Adams, one of the most vocal opponents of the new system, is also one of the most powerful physicians in the department. He has been holding private meetings with others, engaging their support in blocking this effort. His negativism is contagious. Even those initially in favor of the new scheduling system are now beginning to question its value.

Other leading surgeons appear to be withdrawing. Dr. Wright, for example, publicly says little about the new system, but he has failed to come to the meetings you have scheduled to discuss the system's value and how it will work. In addition, surgeons in his group appear to be scheduling more of their cases with your major competitor, and their relationships with you and department nurses are becoming strained.

The situation is becoming increasingly uncomfortable. You know you must deal with the differences among your people, but the strong feelings that have been aroused are threatening personal relationships and making it difficult to look at the situation objectively. While you want people to express their individuality and opinions so that you can engage them in developing new options, it also seems important to reconcile these conflicts so that harmonious pursuit of objectives can be restored. As you ponder the situation, you wonder whether there is any value in the current conflict, what its sources are, and what actions to take to make the most of the current opportunities.

Value of Conflict:
Friend to Be Embraced or Curse to Be Avoided?

Picture yourself as part of a management team being judged in terms of the quantity and the quality of solutions you generate. Your group has a member who regularly challenges conclusions and forces others to critically examine both their assumptions and the logic of their arguments. Would this ongoing source of conflict be embraced as a contributing friend or expelled as a troublesome foe?

Research conducted by Boulding[1] demonstrated that groups containing confederates who played this "devil's advocate" role generated more and superior alternative solutions than groups without such an individual. However, when given permission to eliminate one member, high-performance groups consistently expelled their unique competitive advantage because the person made others feel uncomfortable. These results demonstrate a widely shared reaction to conflict: a recognition of its positive impact on outcomes and an acknowledgment that, for many, it is not personally comfortable. While improved decisions can emerge when conflict leads to identification and consideration of alternative solutions, it also breeds dissatisfaction, discomfort, and reduced cooperation. Leaders often recognize the need to embrace conflict to improve decision quality. Nevertheless, conflict in organizations is not always tolerated and rarely encouraged.[2] As a leader, how can you assess whether the benefits will outweigh the consequences resulting from the conflict you are facing?

Too Little or Too Much

Some level of conflict appears to be both inevitable and valuable.[2] Certainly it can enhance the creative identification of alternative solutions, increase understanding among those willing to listen, force assumptions to be clarified, and provide a mechanism for the cathartic airing of emotions.

The efforts of neither Dr. Adams nor Dr. Wright seem to be having these desired effects, however. While each is taking a very different strategy, both seem to be contributing to stress, a decrease in productivity, impaired decision making, poor working relationships, and possible misallocation of resources to a scheduling system that may be doomed to failure without their support. In addition, while Dr. Adams' meetings may be consuming excess time, Dr. Wright's efforts are also contributing to an unpleasant emotional experience as well as ensuring that relevant information is not shared. While the form of resistance each has chosen is different, both are producing a high level of conflict that will have a negative impact on organizational performance and on the way people feel about being in the department.

Obviously, a lack of conflict would not solve the problem. When people follow their leader over the cliff, no matter what, new ideas are seldom generated and old ideas are not effectively reviewed and tested against current demands.[3-5] It has long been recognized that too much agreement among top management is one of the leading causes of business failures. It may matter little whether the absence of conflict results from blind allegiance to a leader, intimidating consequences for nonconformance, excessive homogeneity among department members, or the absence of incentives encouraging effective organizational performance. In all cases, new ideas will be lost, and performance is likely to suffer during rapidly changing times.

As a leader, therefore, it is critical to seek an optimal level of conflict within your organization. Too little conflict can lead to lethargic adherence to the past, poor decisions, and ineffectiveness, potentially destroying your organization. Too much conflict and the crippling impact of dissension can lead to organizational disintegration by destroying relationships, reducing productivity, and souring attitudes, while leading to the loss of critical personnel.[2] The optimal level varies across organizations and depends on both the nature of the conflict and the manner in which it is expressed.

Overt or Covert:
Which Way Would You Like It?

Dr. Adams opposes the new scheduling system, and it isn't hard to find out why. He'll tell anybody what's wrong with it and how it would need to be fixed to gain his support. Dr. Wright has taken a very different approach. While he and his friends say little publicly about their concerns, they regularly discuss them among themselves and are taking the actions necessary to demonstrate their quiet opposition.

Which way would you like to have your conflict—overt or covert? Zero conflict is not an option in our rapidly changing environment. A lack of evident conflict generally means that either you do not yet have their attention or that they see no value in discussing the situation openly. With Dr. Adams' open opposition, you at least know where you stand. While it might be more desirable to receive his open opposition privately in your office, he is providing the information necessary to identify the problems that must be addressed if the scheduling system is to succeed. Just as it is preferable not to ski or drive a car blindfolded, it is also preferable to obtain critical information from those who are upset during conflict.

Issues or Emotions:
Not All Conflicts Are Created Equal

Conflict can affect the quality of decisions made in an organization as well as the degree to which those decisions are accepted and effectively put in place. Both Dr. Adams and Dr. Wright appear to be challenging the quality of the scheduling system decision and thus are making its successful implementation unlikely.

While conflict between your desire to implement this system and their support for other alternatives appears inevitable, the form this conflict takes will affect your chances of success.

Conflict can either be issue based and thus focused on substantive differences in perspectives or emotionally directed in a negatively charged manner at individuals who oppose your views. While both are forms of conflict, they lead to radically different outcomes.

Issue focused conflict generally enhances people's understanding of professional concerns such as incompatible goals or the sharing of scarce resources, allows identification of problems/solutions, and improves the chance of acceptance of decisions. When it is openly shared, relatively high levels of issue-based conflict typically lead to higher performance levels (as shown on curve Z in figure 1, page 271).

Emotional conflict, by contrast, generally leads to feelings of suspicion, resentment, anger, and frustration along with poor decisions, lower levels of decision acceptance, and disruption of group cohesion.[2,6] In addition, when emotional conflict is covert and not openly shared, its negative effects are exacerbated, and even relatively low levels of it can lead to low levels of performance (as shown on curve X in figure 1).

Therefore, as depicted in figure 1, organizations benefit from relatively high levels of overt issue-based conflict but are seriously harmed by even relatively low levels of covert emotionally-based conflict. It is your job as leader during conflict to steer the focus back to openly clarifying the issues involved, generating alternative solutions, and building acceptance for these decisions.

Who and What Are the Sources of Conflict?

Both Dr. Adams and Dr. Wright appear to be sources of significant problems for implementing the new scheduling/patient tracking system. Because they are the visible sources of conflict, it would seem that one would either need to understand their motives or write them off as defects that should be isolated from the system. While the nature of each of these individuals may well contribute to current tensions, broader ways of

Figure 1. Effects of Conflict on Performance

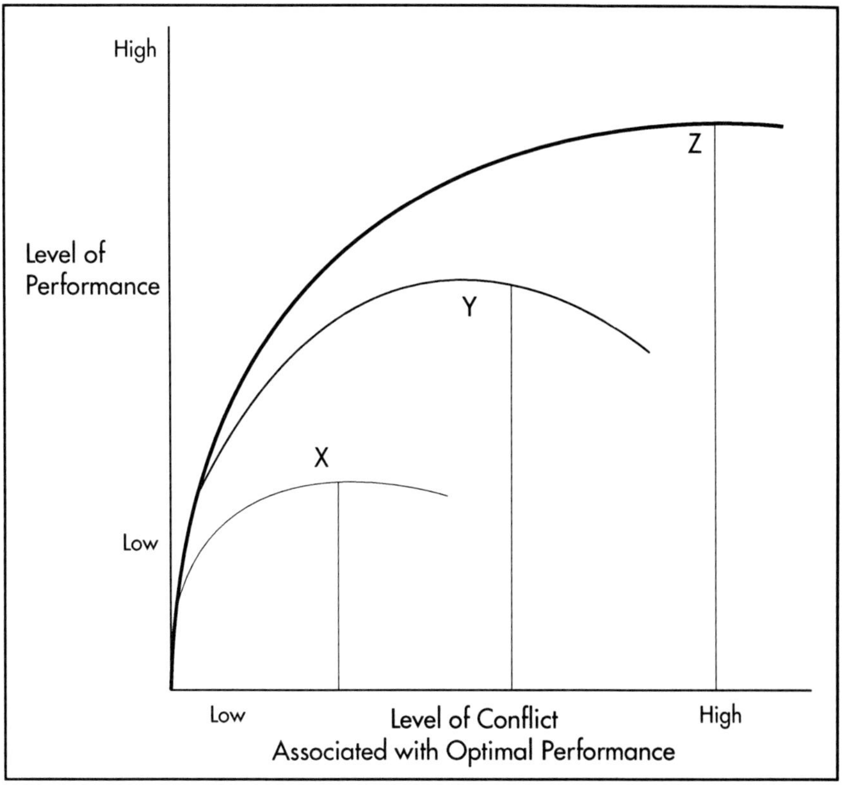

"X" "Y" and "Z" denote optimal level of conflict under three different conditions:
Curve "X" represents mostly covert and emotional conflict
Curve "Y" represents a combination of covert/affective conflict and overt/issue-based conflict
Curve "Z" represents mostly overt and issue-based conflict

thinking about both the sources of and the solutions to conflict are valuable to the effective leader.

Who: Individual Contributions to Conflict

Both personal values and resulting differences in individual goals contribute to conflict within organizations. Sometimes diverse histories and education result in disagreements over ethics, moral considerations, or assumptions about fairness and justice. Such differences may be particularly evident between individuals or groups who have chosen different careers and have been shaped by diverse training. For example, a chief financial officer may be drawn to efficiency and cost containment, while a physician may be more concerned with clinical outcomes and patient satisfaction.

Differences in values and beliefs may lie dormant—unspoken or even unrecognized—until they are confronted by opposing beliefs. My belief that I am underpaid may be only a mild irritation until I go to my class reunion and find peers earning twice my current salary. It is often the presence of organizational conditions (e.g., task relationships, scarce resources, competition) that stir beliefs and move people forward into conflict. The independent, autonomous physician's short-term time perspective, for example, may lie dormant and unnoticed until confronted by the collaborative, participative long-term time perspectives of an administrator during their mutual development of an integrated delivery system.

What: Situational Contributions to Conflict

A common misperception about conflict is that it is primarily personality driven and the result of defective individuals. Two problems exist with this view:

- Our increasingly specialized and diverse work force means that we can't just get rid of people who see the world differently.

- Personality differences are not typically the immediate source of conflict at work. Such differences usually lie dormant until they are triggered by an organizational catalyst.

Organizational catalysts likely to trigger conflict include differential information, incompatible task relationships/incentives, and competition for scarce resources.

> *Differential Information.* To the degree that people have different definitions of the problem, either because they are aware of different pieces of relevant information or because they bring divergent interpretations to the facts that are present, conflict is a likely outcome.[7,8] If there is no communication about these differences, uncertainty and tension increases during rapidly changing times. The resulting anxiety leaves people prone to conflict. While administrators may be expected to view the new scheduling/tracking system as a great way to trim costs by identifying and rectifying process problems, both Dr. Adams and Dr. Wright may see the system as a mechanism for interfering with their ability to make decisions based on patient well-being.

> *Incompatible Task Relationships/Incentives.* To the extent that people in work settings depend on each other to get the job done, separation is not possible. When different authority structures overlap (e.g., surgeons, anesthesiologists, administrators, nurses), tensions naturally rise. To the degree that incentive systems push these groups to pull in inconsistent directions, conflict is a likely outcome. Differences in personal values frequently lie dormant until structural forces come into play and heighten these inconsistencies.

Competition for Scarce Resources. Conflict is more likely to result as the supply of resources becomes noticeably smaller. The threat of loss generates stress and brings old assumptions into conflict with one another. While the debate between administration and both Dr. Adams and Dr. Wright may seem to be about the new scheduling/tracking system, circumstances surrounding that system (e.g., fear of losing resources when the health care resource pool is shrinking) may have much to do with both the level of conflict and the alternative methods these physicians have chosen to deal with their concerns. The normal tendency is to attack individuals who appear to be sources of conflict. It is more effective to understand organizational catalysts and make adjustments. Structural conditions can be more readily manipulated than the values or beliefs individuals hold.

Conflict Management Strategies: Taking Advantage of the Opportunities

While many leaders seek to avoid the discomfort associated with conflict, this strategy may deny them the potentially creative innovation and enhanced performance that can result from opposing viewpoints. There is no one right way to deal with the naturally occurring differences in views that exist within organizations. However, a conscious understanding of alternative approaches to conflict and their consequences is critical to successful leadership. Choices exist for both general strategies and specific action steps fundamental to effectively utilizing the most potentially rewarding of these approaches.

General Strategies

People's responses to conflict can be classified into five general strategies: competing, avoiding, accommodating, compromising, and collaborating.[2,9] These responses can be organized on the basis of the degree to which they are focused on the conflictive issue as opposed to the relationship among conflicting parties, as shown in figure 2, page 274. Accommodating strategies, in the lower right corner of the triangle, focus on the importance of the relationship among involved parties and are intended to satisfy the other parties' concerns. Competing strategies, in the lower left corner of the triangle, focus on the importance of the issue and are intended to ensure that one's own concerns are satisfied. Avoidance and compromise represent differing levels of non-attention to both the relationship and the issue. Collaborating strategies, at the top of the triangle, encompass full attention on both the relationship and the issue.

Competing is a command and control approach designed to overpower other groups, ignore their concerns, and promote one's own position at the expense of others. It can be carried out using one's formal position or

Figure 2. Conflict Resolution Strategies

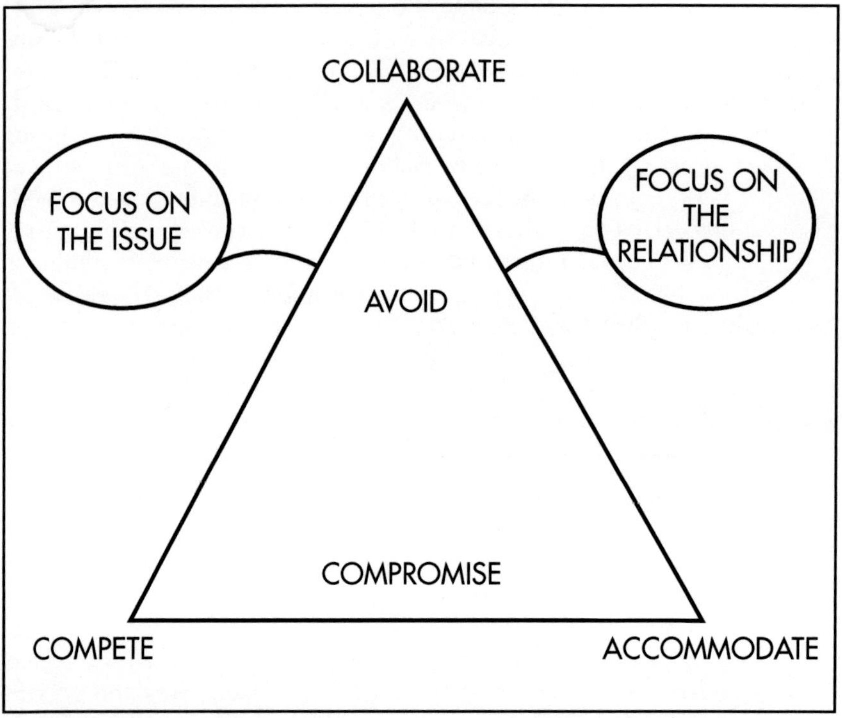

manipulative ploys. While the possibility of behaving as if you are right and getting your way is sometimes appealing, the approach is inappropriate when long-term relationships are important, one's power base is not sufficient to force one's will upon others, or one needs innovative ideas from the other people involved.

If immediate action is required (e.g., business turnaround with limited cash flow, avoidance of an impending clinical crisis) and you have the power to ensure compliance, this strategy may be highly effective. Competing may also be necessary when needed solutions (e.g., downsizing) are likely to be unpopular to some of the people involved or when it is necessary to demonstrate your conviction to those who would take advantage of non-competitive behavior.

These conditions are often not present in professional organizations. For example, in dealing with either Dr. Adams or Dr. Wright, it is unlikely that formal authority exists to impose one's wishes on them. In addition, ignoring their concerns is likely to lead to a worsening of current conditions. The resulting hostility, resentment, and backlash, even if the new scheduling/ tracking system could be imposed, would be detrimental to your future success as a leader.

Accommodating, at the opposite extreme, is an appealing approach for many. By satisfying the other parties' concerns, one appears to be caring for the relationship, building rapport, and creating the right to claim favors at a future time. This strategy may also be appropriate when you recognize that you are wrong, wish to appear reasonable, or lack the power necessary to achieve your desired outcomes.

While the strategy can be highly effective in reconciling differences with minimal time investment, its recurring use in the name of maintaining harmony can result in others' learning to take advantage of you. In addition, all involved may actually lose as a result of not critically appraising issues and selecting optimal solutions if the sources of the conflict are of significant importance to the organization. In the case of the scheduling/tracking system, accommodating the needs of Drs. Adams and Wright would ignore the need for efficiency, cost containment, and enhanced access to medical technology. Accommodating, under such conditions, not only would result in loss of esteem but also would make it more difficult to deal with future issues.

A strategy of *avoiding* conflict has the advantage of saving time and removing oneself from unpleasant circumstances in the short run. This strategy may also be appropriate when conditions suggest that you have no chance of achieving your objectives and that the potential disruption of conflict outweighs any benefits likely to occur. This approach is most useful when the issues are not relevant to organizational performance (e.g., religion, politics, or loyalty to sports teams), no need exists to reach agreement, and the parties involved are not dependent on each other to produce effective performance.

Unfortunately, this approach neglects both one's own needs and those of the other parties involved. Such an approach may be appropriate if the issue and the relationships are unimportant to you and/or circumstances suggest that others who are currently engaged can better handle the conflict. However, assuming that disagreements are inherently bad because of their negative impact on harmony or that this is someone else's problem can have detrimental consequences. Problems don't get solved, and frustration often mounts. As a result, the organization in the long run is in a weaker position to handle ongoing challenges that arise.

Further ongoing avoidance of conflicts regarding the scheduling/tracking system seems impossible. Battle lines have been drawn in different ways by both Dr. Adams and Dr. Wright in response to this administrative imperative. Differences of views must be resolved if confusion, negative feelings, and reduced performance are to be avoided.

Compromising often appears to be an appealing solution that partially avoids both the demands of the issue and the relationships. It allows one to reach an agreement relatively quickly by providing partial satisfaction for all involved, splitting the difference, and spreading the pain. Compromising may be most effective when other approaches have been unsuccessful and it is essential to minimize further disruption in your organization. The approach may also be appropriate when you must reach a solution rapidly, the parties involved are of roughly equivalent power, and all must agree to support the new decision. The regular use of this approach can be counterproductive, however. Conflicts may be postponed and prolonged as each side continues to bemoan its losses and seek further satisfaction of its needs. All involved may simply learn to ask for more in the future so that compromises are closer to their initial desires.

Some form of compromise regarding the scheduling/tracking system may work in the short run (e.g., postpone implementation until further fact finding can occur) if this approach is used to allow time for more effective data gathering and problem solution. Given the importance of the issue to all involved, it is not likely that it will provide a long-term solution to the problem, heal relationships, build trust, or meet the needs of the parties involved on a long-term basis.

Collaboration, the conflict-handling strategy at the top of the triangle in figure 2, focuses on addressing both the issue and the relationship. It is most appropriate when it is important to satisfy the needs of all parties by working through differences and seeking win-win solutions. When both relationships and issues are critical, investing time and energy in this approach will improve future performance.

Under these circumstances, positive conflict resolution strategies are more likely to emerge in face-to-face settings when each of the parties involved has part of the resources (such as information) required to reach a successful solution.[10] When it is important to combine ideas, gain commitment, and improve the capacity to work together on future challenges, a collaborative approach is most likely to channel differences into increasing the range of alternatives, encouraging trust, focusing on issues rather than personalities, and enhancing long-term performance. Given the need to repair relationships, encourage trust, and reach solutions with Drs. Adams and Wright, collaboration appears to be the strategy of choice. In addition to bringing the issues to the surface, it is likely to enhance open as opposed to covert communication and to build a base for resolving both the scheduling/tracking system and future problems.

Collaborative Action Steps

Presuming you wish to resolve an important issue while maintaining or enhancing the relationships among the parties to the conflict and have the time necessary to focus on future success, a collaborative approach seems most appropriate. A number of collaborative action steps are important to the effective implementation of this strategy:

1. Create a context for success.
2. Embrace the conflict.
3. Encourage communication and trust.
4. Clarify critical issues.
5. Work within other people's perspectives.
6. Clarify processes to be followed.
7. Protect and enhance relationships.
8. Ensure support, follow-up, and commitment.

Create a Context for Success (versus focusing on the problem). A leader's job is to create circumstances in which people will choose to come forward, contribute their ideas, and work to achieve mutually agreed-to solutions to conflict situations. Such conditions demand a mutual understanding of where the organization and its members can go as a result of reconciling this conflict and why they should wish to participate in these outcomes. The presence of goals that cannot be achieved without working together provides a framework of common objectives that inspires searching for potential solutions.

Beyond knowing where you might go, it is also essential that people understand why you are going there if they are to be energized to resolve conflict and work together to produce these future outcomes. Describing the future in terms of the individual benefits to be achieved or of the consequences of failure is important in focusing people's attention on the need for reconciling differences. Making these descriptions personal (e.g., impact on their career, earnings, power, prestige) energizes people toward action.

Embrace the Conflict (versus punishing those who verbalize differences). As noted above, most people intellectually assent to the value of conflict while behaviorally avoiding it to the best of their ability. Not only is conflict unpleasant for most of us, but also it violates our basic desire to be nice and not create pain and discomfort for others.

Without leadership intervention, people will typically avoid open expression of conflictive concerns to those who they know will disagree. In order to embrace conflict and encourage others to engage in the pursuit of mutually acceptable solutions, it is important that a leader openly acknowledge that the conflict exists. If steps are not taken to encourage acknowledgment of concerns, the conflict strategies pursued by Dr. Wright will most likely continue. Under these conditions, people are not involved in a process designed to find mutually agreeable solutions. As a result, productivity will suffer and relationships will become increasingly strained.

Encourage Communication and Trust (versus repeatedly being logical, telling people they don't understand, and pushing harder). Abraham Lincoln said, "When I am getting ready to reason with a man, I spend one-third of my time thinking about myself and what I am going to say, and two-thirds thinking about him and what he is going to say."[11] While it is not necessary to ignore your own position, it is critical to put yourself in others' shoes/ heads if you are going to get to mutually acceptable solutions. The ability to see the situation as others do, while difficult, is essential to conflict resolution. Others will believe their views are right just as strongly as you believe yours are right. These views are usually based on prior learning and assumptions, not on the facts involved in the situation.

Trust cannot be demanded or required. The building of trust and a shared understanding of reality involves listening in order to understand rather than telling over and over again how you see things. The building of trust requires an investment in demonstrating understanding and respect for the views of others involved in the conflict. It involves active listening, using open-ended inquiries to elicit further information, and accepting what others have to say while probing for additional clarification.

Active listening and inquiry into the concerns of Dr. Adams and Dr. Wright are essential to beginning to build a bridge that involves them in the process of identifying acceptable solutions to the current scheduling/tracking conflict. You've been hearing Dr. Adams willingly express his ideas, but it will be important to demonstrate your commitment to understanding and then clarifying potential solutions to meet the full range of challenges faced. Having demonstrated your understanding of Dr. Adams' views and your willingness to build them into revisions of the planned systems, you will have increased the likelihood of his being willing to examine outcomes you must produce and engage with you in the development of creative means of reaching these ends.

Dr. Wright has demonstrated the desire for a less open approach, and it may therefore be necessary to create anonymous processes for gathering information about his concerns regarding the scheduling/tracking system. Through the use of anonymous surveys, third-party interviewers, or electronic question and answer systems, one may gather initial information from Dr. Wright and others who have concerns.

Clarify Critical Issues (versus pointing out why they are wrong and you are right). Frustration arises when participants are focused on different aspects of a conflict. For example, administration may be primarily concerned about the goals to be achieved by the new scheduling/tracking system; Drs. Adams and Wright may be much more interested in discussing the methods to be used in achieving those goals. It is important to clarify the issues as the two parties see them.

By managing the discussion effectively, a leader can move the focus toward the issues and away from personality clashes. Maintaining attention on issues rather than on personalities shifts the conversation to descriptive rather than judgmental issues. For example, attention focused on reducing the duration of emergency department visits will be more productive than complaints regarding the slowness of those performing laboratory tests. The former approach allows you to identify process problems while the latter will create defensiveness and an inability to communicate in a manner that generates innovative solutions.

Work within Other People's Perspectives (versus focusing on specific demands). Focusing on specific demands minimizes the likelihood of successfully resolving conflicts. In contrast, coming to understand each party's reasons behind his or her demands—what is really at stake for the person—opens up the possibility of finding creative solutions.

Once you better understand the interests of the parties involved, and they feel understood, brainstorming ways to satisfy all of the needs involved becomes a possible strategy. When a demand is placed before you, it may be appropriate to ask what that demand would get the person that he or she really wants. While it is clear that Dr. Adams and Dr. Wright are upset regarding the new scheduling/tracking system and opposed to its implementation, little has been done to date to clarify the critical issues involved. Until that step is taken, the likelihood of reconciling the conflicts remains low.

Clarify the Process to Be Followed (versus doing the same thing over and over and hoping for a different result). One of the best predictors of future behavior is past behavior. When one is unhappy with the outcomes produced by past behavior, it is usually wise to try something new. While you may hope that others will change their behaviors, taking the lead in reconciling conflict necessitates that you alter your own behavior patterns first. For example, to the degree that the situation continues to be emotionally entangled and based on positions, it may be valuable to suggest the use of objective criteria. Progress may be made through a discussion of what standards could be used or what data could be collected to clarify which of the opposing proposals is most likely to be successful. The conversation may then shift from a focus on getting "what I want" to a focus on deciding what makes the most sense given the agreed-to criteria.

If it has become clear that a disagreement is over facts, progress may be made through validating existing data or developing additional information regarding which of the alternatives best meets the agreed-to criteria. Alternatively, in a situation in which righteous indignation about the moral correctness of values is at stake, it may be useful to move from abstractions to a description of what the values mean in operational terms. Because the same words and concepts mean different things to different people, the process of clarification can lead to a deepened understanding and the possibility of mutually acceptable solutions

For example, initial managerial reactions to a further 10% budget cut demanded by the CEO of a large payer organization included disbelief, frustration, and accusations regarding the unreasonableness of her demands. Hadn't their departments all made several prior cuts in recent years? Were their cost figures not among the best in the industry? Certainly they could not again be expected to turn out the same work with yet a further reduction in resources. However, as these managers began to better understand their leader's plans, they realized that she did not intend that they simply do the same work with fewer people. In fact, what she really wanted was that they further enhance their competitive position by first clarifying what their customers really wanted from the organization. Some services would have to be discontinued, so find out the ones that were most important to the customer. Secondly they needed to reconsider how they could best produce these services—they might need to require less sign-off signatures to make a change or they may have to reduce some layers of management As the process of joint clarification progressed, all involved became more interested in developing the mutually-acceptable solutions required to ensure their ongoing future success.

Protect and Enhance Relationships (versus focusing on getting what you want at any cost). Crisis offers you the opportunity to redefine, through your behavior, how you will do things from this point forward. While words about involvement, listening, and participative decision making are interesting, a leader's behavior during crises speaks far more loudly regarding commitment to these issues. If conflict is to be transformed into problem solving, people's feelings, interests, and general well-being must be protected in the process. By looking for ways to meet their needs and suggesting areas in which parties can make concessions of value to others with little impact on themselves, steps can be taken toward further establishing conditions of caring and trust. For maximum impact, a leader may have to go beyond keeping parties informed about progress and challenges and take the lead in being vulnerable if others are to do the same. This may involve recognizing publicly your contribution to current problems and taking steps to demonstrate your commitment to correcting past inadequacies. Behaviors such as open communication and demonstrating concern for employees, for example, have been found to be positively associated with enhancing trust.[12]

It may be, for example, that Dr. Adams and Dr. Wright, having witnessed your prior refusal to consider their views regarding other issues, have come to conclude that it is useless to engage in a dialogue with you regarding the new scheduling/tracking system. If so, it may be necessary for you to recognize with each of them that you now see the consequences of your prior behavior. In addition, genuine interest in repairing the situation can best be demonstrated by your taking actions to implement some of the suggestions that they have previously provided.

For example, the senior executive of an HMO had consistently refused to provide the funds needed to invest in medical technology physicians had requested for several of the organization's clinics. As conflict about a diversity of issues continued to escalate, he finally chose to acknowledge (at a medical staff meeting) that he regretted the impact of his prior refusals on his relationship with the medical staff, that he now recognized the wisdom of their request, and that money would be made available that week to invest in the requested technology. While other sensitive issues still remained to be addressed, his actions did much to open the door to additional follow-up conflict resolution conversations.

Ensure Support, Follow Up, and Commitment (versus hoping for the best). The appearance of agreement can leave a leader so relieved that final steps in reconciling the conflict are overlooked. It is essential to verify that all parties have a common understanding of their commitments to specific actions. Beyond simply settling for their verbal assent to your summary, it is important to establish mechanisms for follow up. Benchmarks and specific time lines for measuring progress will make the plan tangible and will ensure accountability. While it may be important to encourage flexibility and to adjust the plan to meet emerging circumstances, original agreements regarding measures of success help people recognize that they are agreeing to the same thing.

If benchmarks are not achieved and if Dr. Adams or Dr. Wright continue with their current course of action with respect to agreed-to adjustments, it is necessary to demonstrate your commitment to the agreed-to decisions. If you fail to do this, others will recognize that the scheduling/tracking agreements, as well as other organizational arrangements, have low credibility and are subject to arbitrary change. The lack of consequences for violating agreed-to plans will lead to a lower state of harmony and productivity than existed prior to the conflict. Clarity regarding consequences of not supporting the agreed-to objectives is an essential part of this last step in successfully resolving conflict. Such consequences, if they occur, will not be seen as arbitrary impositions. They will be recognized as a choice made by those who did not keep their agreements.

Clearly, the processes followed by Dr. Adams (e.g., holding private meetings to engage others in blocking the effort) or Dr. Wright (e.g., withdrawal from the situation) are not ideal vehicles for reaching mutually acceptable solutions. Progressing with them through the steps outlined above can create a context and understanding in which new processes can be put into place.

References

1. Boulding, K. "Further Reflections on Conflict Management." In Kahn, R., and Boulding, E., Editors, *Power and Conflict in Organizations*. New York, N.Y.: Basic Books, 1964.

2. Rahim, M. A. *Managing Conflict in Organizations* 3rd ed. London: Quorum Books. 2001

3. Fiol, C. M. & O'Connor, E. J. "Waking up! Mindfulness in the face of bandwagons." *Academy of Management Review* 28(1):54-70, Jan. 2003.

4. O'Connor, E. J. & Fiol, C. M. "Diving into white lightning: Herd behaviors in group practices." *MGMA Connexion* 2(9):22-4, Oct. 2002.

5. O'Connor, E. J. & Fiol, C. M. Mindful over mindless: Learning to think like an entrepreneur. *The Physician Executive* 28(4):18-23, July-Aug. 2002.

6. Nugent, P. S. Managing conflict: Third-party interventions for managers. *Academy of Management Executive* 16(1):139-54, Feb. 2002.

7. Fiol, C. M. & O'Connor, E. J. When hot and cold collide in radical change processes: Lessons from community development. *Organization Science* 13(5):532-46, Sept.-Oct. 2002.

8. O'Connor, E. J. & Fiol, C. M. When hot and cold collide: Riding the spirals of emotions and logic. *The Physician Executive* 28(6):18-21, Nov.-Dec. 2002.

9. Whetten, D., and Cameron, K. *Developing Managerial Skills*. Glenview, Ill.: Scott, Foresman, and Company, 1995.

10. Zornoza, A, Ripoll, P, & Peiro, J. M. Conflict management in groups that work in two different communication contexts: Face-to-face and computer-mediated communication. *Small Group Research* 33(5):481-508, Oct. 2002.

11. Charlton, J., Editor. *The Executive's Quotation Book*. New York: St. Martin's Press, 1983.

12. Korsgaard, M. A., Brodt, S. E., Whitener, E. M. Trust in the face of conflict: The role of managerial trustworthy behavior and organizational context, *Journal of Applied Psychology* 87(2):312-9, April 2002.

Edward J. O'Connor, PhD, is Professor of Management & Health Administration, and **C. Marlena Fiol, PhD**, is Professor of Strategy & Health Administration, University of Colorado at Denver. Both are Principals of the Implementation Institute, Denver.

Chapter 15

How to Get Physician Executive Jobs

by Barbara J. Linney, MA

Physicians who are considering moving from clinical practice into management often ask, "What do you have to do to make the change?" Recruiters and hiring organizations have voiced the base-line requirements described in this chapter regularly over the past 12 years.

Become a Board-Certified Clinician Who Has Practiced 3-5 Years

As a physician executive, you will be working with physicians, in some cases telling them what they can and cannot do. Physicians respect other physicians most for their knowledge of disease and their capacity to take care of patients. Only gradually do they come to respect physician executives for their management skills. They will not take instructions from someone who has not had to cope with an overcrowded schedule, shrinking resources, government regulations, hassles with insurance companies, the threat of malpractice suits, and night call, to name a few of the frustrating realities of being a practicing clinician.

Get Management Experience

Volunteer to serve on and lead committees, such as utilization review, quality assurance, strategic planning, privileging, and credentialing. You can claim all of this service as background experience when you are ready to move more into management. Let people see you doing management activities—working with people, helping groups solve problems, dealing with budgets and schedules. Be excited about new approaches such as a new computer order entry system. Volunteer, in an upbeat, cheerful way, to teach others to use it.

Do what you can to move up in the elected or selected hierarchy of your hospital medical staff. Express interest in becoming chair of your clinical department. Take a job as an elected officer in your medical group or health plan. Get involved in the county medical society, the state medical society, or the American Medical Association.

Some insurance companies and HMOs hire people to do utilization review and quality assurance part time. This can sometimes lead to a full-time job. Even if it doesn't, it is always viewed as valuable management experience. If you know a physician who works on contracts with an HMO, talk to him or her about whom to contact in the organization to try and get the part-time job.

Run short, effective meetings. This is usually the first place people see your leadership skills. If you can't run an effective meeting, they will not think you can do other things well. Create an agenda that people receive ahead of time and that is visible during the meeting. Start on time and stop on time. You can control excessive talkers by having everyone take a minute to write down their thoughts on an agenda topic. First, call on those who always want to talk, give them three minutes and then say, "We need to move to the next person so we can get everyone's opinion." Eventually call on those who resist talking. They will be more forthcoming if they have had a moment to collect their thoughts on paper.

Get Education

Most clinicians need business education if they are going to move into management. I've had several physician executives tell me that they think they didn't make the first cut in the interview process because the other candidates had about the same experience as they did, but they also had master's degrees.

Management education can help you get management experience and perform more effectively if you already have a physician executive position. If you want to serve on the finance committee, you will be a much more valuable member if you have the latest information on the topic. You can take a finance course in a variety of settings. The Physician in Management Seminar of the American College of Physician Executives (ACPE) is an excellent source of training in basic management skills—one day of the week-long seminar is devoted to Finance. There is a four-day live course as well as a CD-Rom and interactive Internet course on financial decision-making.

Be on the alert for informal educational opportunities from other national professional organizations and from local college and universities. Get a master's degree if you have the time and the financial resources. ACPE offers graduate degrees in conjunction with four top universities—an online MBA in conjunction with the University of Massachusetts at Amherst, the Master of Medical Management (MMM) degree, offered in conjunction with Carnegie Mellon University and the University of Southern California, which blends on-campus sessions, independent study, and distance learning, or the Master of Science in Healthcare Quality and Safety Management (MS-HQSM) offered with Thomas Jefferson University.

Be aware, however, that a master's degree will not guarantee that you can get a management job the way the MD or DO guaranteed that you could go practice medicine. You must position yourself to get leadership and management experience at the same time you are getting the degree or after you finish in order to move into a full-time management position.

Fine-Tune Your Interpersonal Communication Skills

A complete assessment of communications skills is provided in Chapter 13. It is important to get out of your office, listen carefully to what people are telling you, and talk to them in a non-arrogant manner. What has become an old adage is true—you need to manage by walking around.

Spend Time on Your Resume

Put together a short, powerful resume, as opposed to a long curriculum vitae. Tell not only where you showed up for work and when (the items usually included in the CV), but also what you accomplished while you were there. Example: Developed a high-technology home care joint venture. Program generated over $1 million in revenue and $250,000 in profit in its first six months.

List your professional experience in reverse chronological order. People want to know most what you have been doing in the past 3-5 years, so lead with these positions in more detail. You can abbreviate the information for prior positions in order to keep the document to three pages.

When you choose items from your curriculum vitae, most likely you will have to add information. True, you worked at St Vincent's Hospital from 1999 to 2002, but what did you do while you were there? Did you help lower costs in the emergency department? Did you help develop clinical guidelines for treating diabetics, resulting in five percent fewer hospitalizations for those patients?

The best resume in the world will not get you a job on its own, but you have to have one that is good enough not to get you thrown out of the job search process. It's networking that gets you the contact who will ask you to send your resume. Then it is the interview that gets you the job or not.

Use Networking Effectively

Get to know more people than you know now. Most people get jobs because they know someone who knows someone who leads to it. Recruiters have told me that 70-90 percent of executive jobs are gotten through networking—not through recruiters.

People have to know who you are and what you can do in order to recommend you for a job. They need to see you tackling problems and working with people. I've known a few people who didn't have all the experience that the hiring organization wished they had, but they got the job because someone knew them and thought they had the qualities it would take to do the job.

First, develop a two-minute summary of yourself, starting with what you are doing now—your interests, competencies, and experiences—and ending with where you want to go. You can write out a script or do it from memory but make sure you can explain what you do and where you're going so that anyone could understand it. You also want to convey excitement and enthusiasm about exploring new opportunities in this personal introduction. (This and many other tips on networking in this chapter are taken from the transcript of the ACPE Cyberforum on "Navigating the Job Search Superhighway" led by Barry Herman, MD.[1])

Once your introduction is firm, develop a list of questions to ask people in your network. "Do you know anyone who may be interested in what I have to offer? Do you know of companies that would have an interest in my skill set? Do you know any recruiters whom I should contact? Do you know others with whom I can network? (The latter question should be used only as a last resort, but it can help identify extraverts who may know just the people you would like to meet.) Notice that these questions avoid asking for a job, because most people may not necessarily know of open positions".[1]

When you are asked about your professional work by someone, you can present your introduction and ask the questions you've developed. Of course, you also want to make it clear you want to learn about the other person so that you establish rapport with the person. Try this method on people that you know, but do not be so selective that you confine your networking to physician friends and acquaintances. Many other casual contacts—the hairdresser, barber, postman, priest, rabbi, etc.—may all have information of value to you.

Increase your visibility by making speeches, writing articles, and serving on committees. Even better is to lead such committees. Make phone calls to people in your network and then call them again to reinforce your interest in them and their knowledge of opportunities. Attend meetings, and talk to people while you are there. Send letters and thank-you notes after encounters with people. Read journals for advertised positions, and monitor job listings on the Internet. Among the Web sites that list employment opportunities are:

- www.acpe.org
- www.ache.org
- www.cejka.com
- www.physicianexecutive.com
- www.tylerandco.com
- www.wittkieffer.com

Achieving visibility involves more work than most people want to do, but few people are able to skip any steps if they wish to be successful.

Get to know the professional recruiters in several search firms that deal regularly in the health care industry. Even if you are not interested in the jobs you see advertised in a journal or on a web site, you can contact recruiters; describe your experience, the kind of job you are looking for, and where you are willing to live; and ask them to keep you in mind for any opportunities that arise. It is always best to make a personal contact before you send your resume. When you know that recruiters will be at association meetings, try to attend so they can put your face with your name.

Pay Attention to Your Executive Image

For interviews, men should wear a dark blue or gray suit, a white shirt, and a conservative tie—stripe, small club, or small paisley. Shoes should look new and over-the-calf socks should be worn. Have a good haircut and trim all wild growing hairs that come with the aging process. Wear an expensive looking watch—not plastic, even if you are an athlete.

Women should wear a dark suit—navy blue, gray, or black. These are power colors and make everyone look their slimmest. Wear a blouse with a neckline high enough that cleavage cannot be seen in any position, medium to low heels, and no dangling earrings or noisy jewelry.

Walk tall, offer a firm but not pain-producing handshake, sit up straight, look alert, and make eye contact 80% of the time.

"How we look will determine the first impression of ourselves, so neat, clean, business-like, punctual, and comfortable count."[1]

Dealing with Recruiters

There are two types of executive search firms—retained and contingency. Retained search firms are paid a fee for their efforts, usually regardless of whether one of their candidates is offered the position or not. Some retained firms spend considerable time getting to know their clients' needs before beginning to seek candidates, spend more time getting to know their candidates and their families, and play a major role in the full scope of recruitment activities.[1]

Contingency firms are paid only when their candidates are placed in jobs. They send your resume to many different organizations. Typically, a retained search firm is the exclusive provider for a search. Several contingency firms may be supplying candidates for the same search.

It is wise to work with many recruiters simultaneously. You can be considered for only one position at a time by any one retained search firm— the retained search firm would look bad if you were selected by two or more of its clients.

Two questions recruiters will ask are: "Will you relocate" and, if so, "What geographic limits do you have?" My experience suggests that it is important to have a "heart to heart" conversation with your significant other before you answer this. It will help you avoid looking at jobs that you ultimately won't accept. On the other hand, if you have little experience, getting the first job may require a move to a less than perfect setting. In management, multiple job changes are the norm.[1]

When considering a position, you conduct the research necessary to answer the following four questions:[1]

- Do you know what the job entails? (You need to obtain job descriptions, discuss the job with human resources personnel if possible, or talk to people who have been in similar positions.)

- Can you do the job? (This question can be answered only after you know what the job entails.)

- Can you do the job the way the employer wants it done? (This question addresses issues of personality/communication style and organizational culture. If you are a big-picture strategist, you need to determine in the interview or through your network if you are being recruited by a detail-oriented tactician.)

- Can you do the job profitably for the employer? (This question relates to issues of productivity and your ability to generate revenue or manage budgets.)

Phone Interview

Every time you pick up the phone, you must be mentally prepared to find someone on the other end of the line who has just started an interview. You may have been extended the courtesy of having someone call to schedule a telephone interview on a specific date and time, but you may also pick up the phone with the TV in the background and lunch in your mouth to find that the interview has already started. It can very difficult for you to get your foot in the door if you don't perform well from the starting gate. You should also try to script potential telephone calls. Anticipate questions and write out your responses. Then read them out loud to be sure they come across as intended on the phone and to implant the questions and your answers in your memory.[1]

Prepare for the Interview

The questions listed below are often asked in physician executive interviews. I recommend that people write the answers to these questions and, if possible, practice them with a friend in front of a video camera before the interview.

1. Tell me briefly what you've been doing since medical school.

2. Why are you looking for a job?

3. Why did you leave your last job?

4. What were your major responsibilities in your last job?

5. What is your greatest strength and your greatest weakness? (Try to couch the weakness in a positive light. Example: "I've been told that sometimes I'm too compassionate with subordinates.")

6. What are your long- and short-term goals? Example of long-term goal: Become CEO of a health care organization. Short-term goal: Develop expertise in utilization management.

7. What are your three greatest accomplishments in your career? Example: Led organization as it changed from being a local health care provider to being a regional provider.

8. What kind of contribution can you make to our company? Example: I believe I can organize and energize the medical staff so that it will feel more supportive of the company's goals.

9. How do you react to criticism?

10. Describe a time when you made a big mistake and how you handled it.

11. Can you give me an example of how you have managed people in the past?

12. How will your spouse feel about your taking this job, about relocating, about your work-related travel? (This question has to be carefully asked by the hiring organization, but it will need to know the answer to it. You would do well to go ahead and offer the information at some point in the interview.)

13. Have you ever hired or fired someone?

14. Why do you want a career in management?

15. How would you deal with a physician who is not performing well?

16. Describe your experience with utilization review and quality assurance.

17. How might you bridge the communication gap between physicians and administrators?

18. Can you describe a time when you analyzed a problem, set a goal, created strategies for solving the problem, implemented the plan, and evaluated the results?

Questions you should ask during the interview

Larry Tyler, CEO of Tyler and Company, an executive search firm, recommends that some of the questions you ask be the same for everyone with whom you meet.[2] Here are some examples of such questions:

- What is it like to work for _____, the CEO, the hiring manager?

- What do you like about working here?

- What would you expect by the end of the first six months?

- How many people have been in this role in the past five years?

- Can I talk to the person who was in this role?

Check for inconsistencies in the responses to these questions and then decide if they matter to you. If the hiring manager says he is a big-picture person, but the COO says he checks on every detail, pay attention to what the majority of respondents say and then decide if your style could mesh with the hiring manager's enough for you to succeed with the organization.

When interviewing with executive directors, CEOs, CFOs, and other business types, even recruiters, don't project the attitude that you have implicit knowledge of all disciplines just because you have a medical degree. You won't get beyond the recruiter if you project a bad impression and he or she thinks you are arrogant.[1]

It is unwise to underestimate the power of social graces in the recruitment process. A candidate who makes a scene during a social event, fails to show his or her human side, or demonstrates negativity or whining will be the loser. Candidates can also get too loose. Be careful about alcohol consumption. A loose tongue can sink a candidacy.[1]

Be Respectful to Everyone

You should behave as if every person with whom you come in contact during a job search can influence the hiring decision. One hiring manager gets regular feedback from an administrative assistant, who lets the manager know how candidates treat members of the manager's staff, how prompt they are in replying, how difficult they are. Candidates who notice that the assistant provides the manager with great service and act on that knowledge get extra points.[1]

Negotiating Your Contract

You won't get everything you want when negotiating a contract, so decide the items that are most important to you. Put all the contract items in a prioritized list and be willing to give up some things at the bottom of the list. Decide which items you have to have or you will not take the job. Regarding the salary for the position, the organization should bring up the issue of money or the recruiting firm may already have told you the salary range.

Remember that you are trying to establish a long-term relationship. Don't be greedy and nit picking. If you make people angry during negotiations, they will not be looking forward to your first day at work. On the other hand, if you don't ask for something you want, you don't have a chance of getting it. Try to find a happy medium. You can ask a lawyer to go over your contract, but don't use the phrase, "My lawyer says…."during the negotiations. That almost always creates ill will. To be sure that your concerns are covered adequately, use a lawyer in the state you are going to, not in the one in which you presently live. This advice is based on the variance in state laws on employment issues.

Consider the following points when negotiating a contract:

Performance Evaluation
• How will your performance be evaluated?

Money
• What is the market value for the position for which you are applying? Learn by reading compensation surveys and talking to others.

- If compensation equals salary plus bonus, what are the criteria for awarding bonuses?

Benefits offered by most organizations

- Insurance: family health and dental, accident, life, short- and long-term disability
- Retirement plans—details of how long until 100% vested, portability
- Continuing education or tuition reimbursement allowance

Paid time off usually includes the following; ask about the numbers

- Vacation days
- Holidays
- Sick days
- Personal days
- CME days

Relocation package

- Are moving expenses and house hunting trips included?

Professional stature issues

- Will malpractice insurance be necessary and are you paying for it? If not, will you be covered by directors and officers (D&O) insurance, and will the organization compensate you for any additional legal expenses?
- Are you expected to maintain specialty certification? What happens if you lose it? Who pays the expenses of maintaining it?
- Is it important to the organization that you maintain medical licenses and membership in medical societies and specialty organizations? If so, what expenses is it willing to cover?

Written agreement

- Will there be a letter of agreement or a more formal contract?
- Are there restrictive covenants?
- Do you need to have a lawyer review the contract?

Termination issues

- Is there a severance package? (In these days of mergers and acquisitions, a severance package should be negotiated when you take the job, not when you are about to leave it.)[1]
- If you have a non-compete clause, it should not be longer than the months allotted in your severance package.

What If You Are Fired?

"If people were fired one-tenth as often as that fear crosses their minds, few of us would be left at work today. The 'big picture' guidance on the threat of job loss is to keep your work game within your life game. When life is the greater game, you will use work in service to life. For example, you will have savings that could get you through lean financial times. And you will have built your personal power at work by being ready to leave if you must—while hoping that would not be necessary. The big answers to this big 'what if…' are in your preparation long before the moment comes."[3]

Coile and Tyler have a different take on the firing issue.[4] "The chances that you will be between jobs at some point in your career are 100 percent. It is unavoidable. But there are things that you can do to make your job loss as painless as possible.

- *Negotiate a contract up front.* Realizing that you might get the axe, be sure that you have a contract that covers severance arrangements and spells out your benefit considerations. Contracts are quite common, and there shouldn't be any reason that a health care executive would not have one in this day and age. Severance arrangements usually are for at least a year's compensation and benefits.

- *Don't lose your temper.* It is easy to get angry and try to get even by verbally abusing your superior or badmouthing the administration or the board to everyone who will listen. This is bad form and will cause you problems on two fronts. First, the people you are badmouthing may need to be used as a reference. If you have said nasty things about them you can count on a negative reference. Secondly, the people who are going to hire you don't want to hear all the gory details either. They would rather hear what you can do for the organization and see you conduct yourself with dignity.

- *Ask for your wish list quickly.* The best time to negotiate is when the boss or the Board is feeling guilty. The longer an issue is hanging, the harder it is for the employer to accommodate your requests. In your career file (the one with your resume in it), you should have put together a list of things that you would need if you were no longer employed and needed to look for a job—for example, office space, secretarial help, and voice mail. If you haven't done this, you should start when you finish this chapter.

- *Be reluctant to sue your former employer.* You can engage a lawyer to represent you and you can threaten to sue, but never actually file the suit unless the payoff is going to be in the millions. Once a lawsuit becomes public, potential employers will be shy about interviewing you and offering you a job. Many times, the executive's grievance is real and genuine; nevertheless, an out-of-court settlement is the best course to pursue. The most extreme example happened…a CEO [who] sued the hospital board after his dismissal. He actually won his case, receiving a judgment of $1. He never got another hospital CEO opportunity during the rest of his career.

- *Tell your family as soon as possible.* Some executives are so upset about their situation that they are reluctant to tell their families that they have lost their positions. This is unfortunate, because the family can offer great support to an out-of-work executive. Additionally, they need to know that the situation has changed and be able to plan accordingly. A good cry with a willing group of supporters can get a lot of emotion out of the way and clear the attitudinal decks for the beginnings of a job search.

- *Take only a brief vacation.* Some executives decide that a sabbatical is in order immediately after a firing and take six months off before ever beginning a job search. This is a bad idea. While there is probably going to be some need to reduce the stress level, take only a week vacation, then get your job search started quickly. You may need to prepare the house for sale. You need to get your resume updated and start calling people while your skills, attitude, and work history are still fresh. Take another vacation right after you are re-employed and before you report to work.

- *Consider a temporary assignment.* Those of us in health care are familiar with locum tenens physicians. Well, there are lots of opportunities for temporary executive assignments. Because of the downsizing in health care, there are fewer executives in the executive suite. Therefore, each executive that is left is very important to the workings of an organization. It is common now for the organization to employ a temporary executive while it seeks a permanent replacement or contemplates the future of the position. Sometimes these executives are eventually employed on a permanent basis. Taking a temporary job keeps you active in the field with money coming in.

- *Be prepared to be re-employed by your former employer.* As strange as it may sound, sometimes positions are eliminated and then the employee is re-employed on a contract or permanent basis. I have several friends at IBM who had this happen to them. Maybe there is a big project like JCAHO accreditation coming up or maybe someone else in the organization left unexpectedly. If you have conducted yourself professionally, you will be eligible for rehire—another reason not to sue your employer.

- *Keep a positive attitude.* Maybe getting fired is the best thing that ever happened to you. Perhaps you hated your job or your circumstances.

Perhaps you were underutilized and capable of bigger things. The stories I have heard from candidates about fortuitous firings are too numerous to list. Some of our greatest leaders in politics, the military, and business have been fired. Winston Churchill, Douglas MacArthur, and Bernie Marcus of Home Depot come immediately to mind. This door may be closing with a bang, but other doors will be opening soon. It has happened to hordes of others and it can happen to you. And if you need cheering up, try www.workingwounded.com, where you can see the gripes of people who hate their jobs and would love to be somewhere else.

Preparing for Change

Entering the world of medical management usually requires changes that the physician and his or her family did not anticipate when he or she became a physician. Here are some issues to think about and talk about with family, friends, and even counselors before you make the leap and afterwards.

Geography/Location

Where are you willing to live? If you say anywhere, recruiters think you haven't thought about it hard enough and certainly haven't talked to your spouse. Many candidates have turned down job offers that have been in the works for months because the spouse said, "I won't go." Some have gone anyway and eventually ended the marriage. Because the physician executive career might require several moves, talk about it now.

Family Concerns

If you convince your spouse to go and then one or both of you are miserable, go to a counselor. I stayed angry for a year after I moved with my pediatrician husband from North Carolina to Florida for him to become a medical director. Then we went to counseling. I spewed forth all that I was upset about and the counselor could restate it in a less inflammatory way. He could describe his point of view, and the counselor could restate it in words I could hear. Then we made some changes where some sacrifices were made for me. I started to work on a PhD in a city 100 miles away. Going to school always made me happier. I left town for 24 hours, and he took care of our grammar school age children.

We should have gone to a counselor after three months of my being miserable.

Health Issues

Some people need to live in warm climates where muscle aches are less pronounced; others don't do well with the pollen production of year-round warm weather. Some like the dry west of Arizona; others the adrenaline-pumping pace of life in a northeastern city. Some cannot bear long dark winters, but others thrive where they can enjoy snow sports for months. Don't dismiss these preferences and think you will be happy anywhere if the job is right.

Lifestyle

What is lifestyle? Here are some examples. My husband listens to classical music everyday, but he does not like to dress up and go to the symphony. He likes to listen to music in his car or in our family room with his shoes off. The existence and quality of the Charlotte symphony do not concern him. For others, it is important to be in a metropolitan area that gives access to a great symphony and other artistic opportunities.

I knew a physician executive who loved horses. He lived in the country and flew his own small plane to work in Dallas every day.

Another couple from Arizona were planning a move to the northeast. After two good interviews, they couldn't figure out why the position didn't seem quite right. They finally realized the sun had not shown any of the days they were in the city for the interviews. They were used to the regular sun of Arizona and decided not to go.

When it comes to lifestyle, only you can decide what you like and don't like. Don't let someone else tell you what yours should be. Be honest with yourself and within reason, try to get those needs met.

Financial Needs

How much money do you need now and in the future? Do you have children to educate, a mortgage? What amount of money will it take to maintain the lifestyle you desire in retirement? Talk to a financial planner who is not trying to sell you something to get the answers to these questions.

Physician executive salaries can be a step up for primary care specialties but are often a step down for other specialties. Can you and your family make the adjustment? Talk about what sacrifices will have to be made and why. If you are bored or, conversely, extremely stressed in your present job, you need to plan for a change and include family members in your thinking processes.

Culture Shock

You need to consider the implications of not being viewed as a clinician any more. Physicians often see you as a traitor who has become one of the "suits." Other administrators think you are still one of the doctors and don't truly understand the need to cut costs. Even if you start your physician executive career as 50 percent clinician and 50 percent management, each group will think you are more loyal to the other. These are over-generalizations, but, if you experience them, you may need to seek support and friends. Many of them may be found when you attend professional meetings with others who are also straddling the fence.

Getting your first physician executive job is harder than getting the second. Once you have had an official title and the experience that goes with it, getting the next one is easier, but it often requires a geographic move. Many physician executives find the required changes to a new job exciting and challenging. Glenn Swogger puts it this way, "Whenever we make a change or embark on a new path, we are in a sense betting on ourselves. We are betting on our perseverance, on our faith in the future, on our ability to trust the love and support of others whom we need to achieve our goals, and on the value of what we do. In that sense, a transition can test and develop the finest qualities that we have."[5]

References

1. ACPE Cyberforum on *"Navigating the Job Search Superhighway"* led by Barry Herman, MD, Nov. 15-Dec. 17,1999.

2. Personal communication, Larry Tyler, CEO of Tyler and Company, Atlanta, Ga.

3. Bellman, G. *Getting Things Done When You Are Not in Charge.* San Francisco, Calif.: Berrett-Koehler Publishers, Inc., 2001.

4. Coile, R., and Tyler, L. "Falling from the Top: The Fired Physician Executive." *Physician Executive* 26(4):12-18, July-Aug. 2000.

5. Swogger, G., MD. "Transition and Its Discontents." *Physician Executive.* 14(5) 14-17, Sept.-Oct. 1988.

Barbara J. Linney, MA, is Vice President of Career Development for the American College of Physician Executives, Tampa, Florida.

CPSIA information can be obtained at www.ICGtesting.com
Printed in the USA
BVOW052355311011

274962BV00001B/11/P